XINGYIQUAN

Theory, Applications, Fighting Tactics and Spirit

XINGYIQUAN

Theory, Applications,
Fighting Tactics and Spirit

形 意 拳

Liang, Shou-Yu & Dr. Yang, Jwing-Ming

YMAA Publication Center
Wolfeboro, NH USA

YMAA Publication Center
Main Office:
    PO Box 480
    Wolfeboro, New Hampshire, 03894
    800-669-8892 • info@ymaa.com • www.ymaa.com

ISBN: 9780940871410 (print)
ISBN: 9781594391781 (ebook)
ISBN: 9781594394218 (hardcover)

20240118

Edited by James O'Leary
Cover design by Richard Rossiter

Publisher's Cataloging in Publication

(Prepared by Quality Books Inc.)

Liang, Shou-Yu, 1943-
    Xingyiquan : theory, applications, fighting tactics, &
spirit / Liang, Shou-Yu and Yang, Jwing-Ming.— 2nd ed.
    p. cm
    Includes bibliographical references and index.
    LCCN: 2002108593
    ISBN: 0-940871-41-6

    1. Martial Arts—China. I. Yang, Jwing-Ming 1946-
II. Liang, Shou-Yu, 1943- Hsing yi chuan. III. Title.
GV1100.7.A2L48 2002   796.8'0951

QBI02-200569

Disclaimer:
The authors and publisher of this material are NOT RESPONSIBLE in any manner whatsoever
for any injury which may occur through reading or following the instructions in this manual.
The activities, physical or otherwise, described in this material may be too strenuous or
dangerous for some people, and the reader(s) should consult a physician before engaging in
them.

Printed in USA.

Dedicated to Mr. Liang's Xingyiquan masters:
Master Zheng, Huai-Xian (鄭懷賢) and
Master Wang, Shu-Tian (王樹田).

Also, a Special Dedication to
Mr. Jeffery D.S. Liang (梁德馨) for Sponsoring
Master Liang's Passage to North America.

Romanization of Chinese Words

This book uses the Pinyin romanization system of Chinese to English. Pinyin is standard in the People's Republic of China, and in several world organizations, including the United Nations. Pinyin, which was introduced in China in the 1950's, replaces the Wade-Giles and Yale systems. In some cases, the more popular spelling of a word may be used for clarity.

Some common conversions:

Pinyin	Also Spelled As	Pronunciation
Qi	Chi	chē
Qigong	Chi Kung	chē kŭng
Qin Na	Chin Na	chĭn nă
Jin	Jing	jĭn
Gongfu	Kung Fu	gōng foo
Taijiquan	Tai Chi Chuan	tī jē chüén

For more information, please refer to *The People's Republic of China: Administrative Atlas, The Reform of the Chinese Written Language,* or a contemporary manual of style.

Contents

About the Author

Master Liang, Shou-Yu 梁守渝先生

Master Liang, Shou-Yu was born June 28, 1943 in the city of Chongqing (重慶), Sichuan Province (四川省), China. When he was six he began his training in Qigong (氣功), the art of breathing and internal energy control, under the tutelage of his renowned grandfather, the late Liang, Zhi-Xiang (梁芷箱). He was taught the esoteric skills of the Emei Mountain sect (峨嵋), including Da Peng Qigong (大鵬氣功). When he was eight, his grandfather made special arrangements for him to begin training Emei Wushu (峨嵋武術).

In 1959, as a young boy, Mr. Liang began the study of Chin Na (擒拿) and Chinese Shuai Jiao (摔跤)(Wrestling). From 1960 to 1964 he devoted his attention to the systematic research and practice of Wrestling, Wushu, and other training.

In addition to the advantage of being born to a Wushu family, Mr. Liang also had the chance to come into contact with many of the legendary grandmasters. By the time he was twenty, Mr. Liang had already received instruction from 10 of the most well-known contemporary masters of both Southern and Northern origin, who gladly instructed and inspired this ardent, young man. His curiosity inspired him to learn more than one hundred sequences from many different styles. His study of the martial arts has taken him throughout mainland China, having gone to Henan Province (河南省) to learn Chen style Taijiquan (陳氏太極拳), Hubei Province (湖北省) to learn the Wudang (武當) system, and Hunan Province (湖南省) to learn the Nan Yue (南嶽) system.

With his wealth of knowledge, Mr. Liang was inspired to compete in martial arts competitions, in which he was many times a noted gold medalist. During his adolescence, Mr. Liang won titles in Chinese wrestling (Shuai Jiao), various other martial arts, and weight lifting.

As he grew older, through and beyond his college years, his wide background in various martial arts helped form his present character, and led him to achieve a high level of martial skill. Some of the styles he concentrated on include the esoteric Emei system (峨嵋), Shaolin (少林), Long Fist (Changquan, 長拳), Praying Mantis (Tang Lang, 螳螂), Cuo Jiao (戳腳), Xingyi (形意), Bagua (八卦), Taiji (太極), Liu He Ba Fa (六合八法), Shuai Jiao (摔跤), Chin Na (擒拿), vital point striking, many weapons systems, and several kinds of internal Qigong.

Mr. Liang received a university degree in biology in 1964. However, it was a time of political turmoil, and because of his bourgeois family background the Communist government sent him to a remote, poverty stricken village to teach high school. However, despite this setback, Mr. Liang began to organize Wushu teams in the local community, and he trained numerous farmer-students in Wushu and wrestling.

Then came a disastrous time in modern Chinese history. During the years of the Cultural Revolution (1966-1974)(文化大革命), all forms of martial arts and Qigong were suppressed. Because he came from a bourgeoisie family, Mr. Liang was vulnerable to the furious passions and blind madness of the revolutionaries. To avoid conflict with the red guards, he gave up his teaching position. However, he then used this opportunity to tour the various parts of the country to visit and discover great masters in Wushu, and to make friends with people who shared his devotion to and love for the art. Mr. Liang went through numerous provinces and large cities, visiting especially the many renowned and revered places where Wushu originated, was developed and polished. Among the many places he visited were Emei Mountain (峨嵋山), Wudang Mountain (武當山), Hua Mountain (華山), Qingcheng Mountain (青城山), Chen's village (陳家溝) in Henan (河南), the Cangzhou Territory (滄州) in Hebei Province (河北省), Beijing (北京), and Shanghai (上海). In eight years he made many Wushu friends and met many great masters, and his mastery of the techniques and philosophy of the art grew to new horizons.

At the end of the Cultural Revolution, the Chinese government again began to support the martial arts and Qigong, including competition. There was a general consensus that they should organize and categorize the existing martial and internal arts. Research projects were set up to search out the old masters who remained alive, select their best techniques, and organize their knowledge. It was at this time that the Sichuan government appointed Mr. Liang as a coach for the city, the territory, and the province. So many of his students were among the top martial artists of China that in 1978 he was voted one of the top national coaches since 1949. He also received acclamation from the People's Republic of China Physical Education and Sports Commissions. After that he often served as judge in national competitions.

After the Cultural Revolution, despite his many official duties Mr. Liang continued to participate actively in competitions at the provincial and national level. Between 1974 and 1981 he won numerous medals, including four gold medals. His students also performed superbly in national and provincial open tournaments, winning many medals. Many of these students have now become professional Wushu coaches or college Wushu instructors themselves. Other students have become Wushu trainers in the armed forces, or have become movie actors in Wushu pictures. In 1979, Mr. Liang received several appointments, including membership in the Sichuan Chapter of the China National Wushu Association, and an executive membership of the Wushu Coaches Committee.

1981 marked a new era in the course of Mr. Liang's life when he first visited Seattle, a coastal city in the state of Washington in the U.S.A. His art impressed every one of the Wushu devotees immediately, and the Wushu and Taiji Club of the Students Association of the University of Washington retained him as a Wushu Coach. At the same time, Mr. Liang was giving lessons in the Taiji Association in Seattle. In the following year, Mr. Liang went north to Vancouver, Canada, and was appointed Taiji Coach by the Villa Cathy Care Home. The same year, he was appointed Honorary Chairman and Head Coach by the North American Taiji Athletic Association.

In 1984, Mr. Liang was appointed Chairperson and Wushu Coach by the School of Physical Education of the University of British Columbia. In 1985, Mr. Liang was elected coach of the First Canadian National Wushu Team, which was invited to participate in the First International Wushu Invitational Tournament which took place in Xian (西安), China. Competing against teams from 13 other countries, the Canadian team won second place.

In 1985, Mr. Liang was again elected coach of the Second Canadian National Wushu Team, which competed in the Second International Wushu Invitational Tournament held in the city of Tianjin (天津), China. A total of 28 countries participated. This time, the Canadian team earned more medals than any other country except the host country. Mr. Liang's role and achievements were reported in 14 newspapers and magazines throughout China, and the performances and demonstrations of the Canadian Team and Mr. Liang were broadcasted on the Sichuan television station.

Mr. Liang has not limited his contributions to Wushu only to Vancouver, Canada. He has also given numerous lectures and demonstrations to Wushu professionals and instructors in the United States, including instructors and professionals from such disciplines as Karate, Taiji, and others. Students in such cities as Houston, Denver, Boston, and New York have benefited from Mr. Liang's personal touch. Mr. Liang has also judged in the National Wushu Tournament in the U.S.A. Mr. Liang has also produced an instructional video program teaching Liangong Shi Ba Fa Qigong (練功十八法氣功) in conjunction with the Chinese National Qigong Institute.

About the Author

Dr. Yang, Jwing-Ming, Ph.D. 楊俊敏博士

Dr. Yang, Jwing-Ming was born on August 11th, 1946, in Xinzhu Xian (新竹縣), Taiwan (台灣), Republic of China (中華民國). He started his Wushu (武術)(Gongfu or Kung Fu, 功夫) training at the age of fifteen under the Shaolin White Crane (Bai He, 少林白鶴) Master Cheng, Gin-Gsao (曾金灶)(1911-1976). Master Cheng originally learned Taizuquan (太祖拳) from his grandfather when he was a child. When Master Cheng was fifteen years old, he started learning White Crane from Master Jin, Shao-Feng (金紹峰), and followed him for twenty-three years until Master Jin's death.

In thirteen years of study (1961-1974) under Master Cheng, Dr. Yang became an expert in the White Crane Style of Chinese martial arts, which includes both the use of barehands and of various weapons such as saber, staff, spear, trident, two short rods, and many other weapons. With the same master he also studied White Crane Qigong (氣功), Qin Na (or Chin Na, 擒拿), Tui Na (推拿) and Dian Xue massages (點穴按摩), and herbal treatment.

At the age of sixteen, Dr. Yang began the study of Yang Style Taijiquan (楊氏太極拳) under Master Kao, Tao (高濤). After learning from Master Kao, Dr. Yang continued his study and research of Taijiquan with several masters and senior practitioners such as Master Li, Mao-Ching (李茂清) and Mr. Wilson Chen (陳威伸) in Taipei (台北). Master Li learned his Taijiquan from the well-known Master Han, Ching-Tang (韓慶堂), and Mr. Chen learned his Taijiquan from Master Zhang, Xiang-San (張祥三). Dr. Yang has mastered the Taiji barehand sequence, pushing hands, the two-man fighting sequence, Taiji sword, Taiji saber, and Taiji Qigong.

When Dr. Yang was eighteen years old he entered Tamkang College (淡江學院) in Taipei Xian to study Physics. In college he began the study of traditional Shaolin Long Fist (Changquan or Chang Chuan, 少林長拳) with Master Li, Mao-Ching at the Tamkang College Guoshu Club (淡江國術社)(1964-1968), and eventually became an assistant instructor under Master Li. In 1971 he completed his M.S. degree in Physics at the National Taiwan University (台灣大學), and then served in the Chinese Air Force from 1971 to 1972. In the service, Dr. Yang taught Physics at the Junior Academy of the Chinese Air Force (空軍幼校) while also teaching Wushu. After being honorably discharged in 1972, he returned to Tamkang College to teach Physics and resumed study under Master Li, Mao-Ching. From Master Li, Dr. Yang learned Northern Style Wushu, which includes both barehand (especially kicking) techniques and numerous weapons.

In 1974, Dr. Yang came to the United States to study Mechanical Engineering at Purdue University. At the request of a few students, Dr. Yang began to teach Gongfu (Kung Fu), which resulted in the foundation of the Purdue University Chinese Kung Fu Research Club in the spring of 1975. While at Purdue, Dr. Yang also taught college-credited courses in Taijiquan. In May of 1978 he was awarded a Ph.D. in Mechanical Engineering by Purdue.

In 1980, Dr. Yang moved to Houston to work for Texas Instruments. While in Houston he founded Yang's Shaolin Kung Fu Academy, which was eventually taken over by his disciple Mr. Jeffery Bolt after moving to Boston in 1982. Dr. Yang founded Yang's Martial Arts Academy (YMAA) in Boston on October 1, 1982.

In January of 1984 he gave up his engineering career to devote more time to research, writing, and teaching. In March of 1986 he purchased property in the Jamaica Plain area of Boston to be used as the headquarters of the new organization, Yang's Martial Arts Association. The organization has continued to expand, and, as of July 1st 1989, YMAA has become just one division of Yang's Oriental Arts Association, Inc. (YOAA, Inc.).

In summary, Dr. Yang has been involved in Chinese Wushu since 1961. During this time, he has spent thirteen years learning Shaolin White Crane (Bai He), Shaolin Long Fist (Changquan), and Taijiquan. Dr. Yang has more than thirty-two years of instructional experience: seven years in Taiwan, five years at Purdue University, two years in Houston, Texas, and eighteen years in Boston, Massachusetts.

In addition, Dr. Yang has also been invited to offer seminars around the world to share his knowledge of Chinese martial arts and Qigong. The countries he has visited include Argentina, Austria, Barbados, Belgium, Bermuda, Botswana, Canada, Chile, England, France, Germany, Holland, Hungary, Ireland, Italy, Latvia, Mexico, Poland, Portugal, Saudi Arabia, Spain, South Africa, Switzerland, and Venezuela.

Since 1986, YMAA has become an international organization, which currently includes 51 schools located in Argentina, Belgium, Canada, Chile, England, France, Holland, Hungary, Ireland, Italy, Poland, Portugal, South Africa, Spain, Venezuela and the United States. Many of Dr. Yang's books and videotapes have been translated into languages such as French, Italian, Spanish, Polish, Czech, Bulgarian, Russian, Hungarian, and Iranian.

Dr. Yang has published twenty-seven other volumes on the martial arts and Qigong:

1. Shaolin Chin Na; Unique Publications, Inc., 1980.
2. Shaolin Long Fist Kung Fu; Unique Publications, Inc., 1981.
3. Yang Style Tai Chi Chuan; Unique Publications, Inc., 1981.
4. Introduction to Ancient Chinese Weapons; Unique Publications, Inc., 1985.
5. Qigong for Health and Martial Arts; YMAA Publication Center, 1985.

6. Northern Shaolin Sword; YMAA Publication Center, 1985.

7. Tai Chi Theory and Martial Power; YMAA Publication Center, 1986.

8. Tai Chi Chuan Martial Applications; YMAA Publication Center, 1986.

9. Analysis of Shaolin Chin Na; YMAA Publication Center, 1987.

10. Eight Simple Qigong Exercises for Health; YMAA Publication Center, 1988.

11. The Root of Chinese Qigong—The Secrets of Qigong Training; YMAA Publication Center, 1989.

12. Muscle/Tendon Changing and Marrow/Brain Washing Chi Kung—The Secret of Youth; YMAA Publication Center, 1989.

13. Hsing Yi Chuan—Theory and Applications; YMAA Publication Center, 1990.

14. The Essence of Taiji Qigong—Health and Martial Arts; YMAA Publication Center, 1990.

15. Qigong for Arthritis; YMAA Publication Center, 1991.

16. Chinese Qigong Massage—General Massage; YMAA Publication Center, 1992.

17. How to Defend Yourself; YMAA Publication Center, 1992.

18. Baguazhang—Emei Baguazhang; YMAA Publication Center, 1994.

19. Comprehensive Applications of Shaolin Chin Na—The Practical Defense of Chinese Seizing Arts; YMAA Publication Center, 1995.

20. Taiji Chin Na—The Seizing Art of Taijiquan; YMAA Publication Center, 1995.

21. The Essence of Shaolin White Crane; YMAA Publication Center, 1996.

22. Back Pain—Chinese Qigong for Healing and Prevention; YMAA Publication Center, 1997.

23. Ancient Chinese Weapons; YMAA Publication Center, 1999.

24. Taijiquan—Classical Yang Style; YMAA Publication Center, 1999.

25. Tai Chi Secrets of Ancient Masters; YMAA Publication Center, 1999.

26. Taiji Sword—Classical Yang Style; YMAA Publication Center, 1999.

27. Tai Chi Secrets of W«u & Li Styles; YMAA Publication Center, 2001.

28. Tai Chi Secrets of Yang Style, YMAA Publication Center, 2001.

29. Tai Chi Secrets of Wu Style; YMAA Publication Center, 2002.

Dr. Yang has also published the following videotapes:

1. Yang Style Tai Chi Chuan and Its Applications; YMAA Publication Center, 1984.
2. Shaolin Long Fist Kung Fu—Lien Bu Chuan and Its Applications; YMAA Publication Center, 1985.
3. Shaolin Long Fist Kung Fu—Gung Li Chuan and Its Applications; YMAA Publication Center, 1986.
4. Shaolin Chin Na; YMAA Publication Center, 1987.
5. Wai Dan Chi Kung — The Eight Pieces of Brocade; YMAA Publication Center, 1987.
6. The Essence of Tai Chi Chi Kung; YMAA Publication Center, 1990.
7. Qigong for Arthritis; YMAA Publication Center, 1991.
8. Qigong Massage—Self Massage; YMAA Publication Center, 1992.
9. Qigong Massage—With a Partner; YMAA Publication Center, 1992.
10. Defend Yourself 1—Unarmed Attack; YMAA Publication Center, 1992.
11. Defend Yourself 2—Knife Attack; YMAA Publication Center, 1992.
12. Comprehensive Applications of Shaolin Chin Na 1; YMAA Publication Center, 1995.
13. Comprehensive Applications of Shaolin Chin Na 2; YMAA Publication Center, 1995.
14. Shaolin Long Fist Kung Fu—Yi Lu Mai Fu & Er Lu Mai Fu; YMAA Publication Center, 1995.
15. Shaolin Long Fist Kung Fu—Shi Zi Tang; YMAA Publication Center, 1995.
16. Taiji Chin Na; YMAA Publication Center, 1995.
17. Emei Baguazhang 1; Basic Training, Qigong, Eight Palms, and Applications; YMAA Publication Center, 1995.
18. Emei Baguazhang 2; Swimming Body Baguazhang and Its Applications; YMAA Publication Center, 1995.
19. Emei Baguazhang 3; Bagua Deer Hook Sword and Its Applications; YMAA Publication Center, 1995.
20. Xingyiquan—12 Animal Patterns and Their Applications; YMAA Publication Center, 1995.
21. 24 and 48 Simplified Taijiquan; YMAA Publication Center, 1995.
22. White Crane Hard Qigong; YMAA Publication Center, 1997.
23. White Crane Soft Qigong; YMAA Publication Center, 1997.
24. Xiao Hu Yan—Intermediate Level Long Fist Sequence; YMAA Publication Center, 1997.

25. Back Pain—Chinese Qigong for Healing and Prevention; YMAA Publication Center, 1997.
26. Scientific Foundation of Chinese Qigong; YMAA Publication Center, 1997.
27. Taijiquan, Classical Yang Style; YMAA Publication Center, 1999.
28. Taiji Sword, Classical Yang Style; YMAA Publication Center, 1999.
29. Chin Na in Depth—Course One; YMAA Publication Center, 2000.
30. Chin Na in Depth—Course Two; YMAA Publication Center, 2000.
31. San Cai Jian & Its Applications; YMAA Publication Center, 2000.
32. Kun Wu Jian & Its Applications; YMAA Publication Center, 2000.
33. Qi Men Jian & Its Applications; YMAA Publication Center, 2000.
34. Chin Na in Depth—Course Three; YMAA Publication Center, 2001.
35. Chin Na in Depth—Course Four; YMAA Publication Center, 2001.
36. Twelve Routines of Tan Tui; YMAA Publication Center, 2001.
37. Chin Na in Depth—Course Five; YMAA Publication Center, 2002.
38. Chin Na in Depth—Course Six; YMAA Publication Center, 2002.
39. Chin Na in Depth—Course Three; YMAA Publication Center, 2002.
40. Chin Na in Depth—Course Seven; YMAA Publication Center, 2002.
41. Chin Na in Depth—Course Eight; YMAA Publication Center, 2002.
42. Chin Na in Depth—Course Nine; YMAA Publication Center, 2002.
43. Chin Na in Depth—Course Ten; YMAA Publication Center, 2002.

Foreword

Since the 1960's, Chinese martial arts have become more and more popular in the Western world. This is especially true of the internal styles such as Taijiquan (太極拳), Xingyiquan (形意拳), and Baguazhang (八卦掌). This has happened because more and more people are realizing that by practicing these arts they can not only learn effective techniques for self defense, but they can also gain a significant improvement in their health.

This fact is not surprising if you understand that the internal Chinese martial styles are based on Qi theory, and are considered to be part of Qigong (氣功)(internal energy) training. Qi is the Chinese word for the natural energy of the universe. Qigong is the science of this energy, especially as it circulates in the human body. The Chinese have been studying Qi for over four thousand years, and they have learned how to apply their knowledge of this energy to meditation and to certain types of movement in order to improve physical and mental health and increase longevity. They have found that Qi theory and principles can also be used to increase muscular power to a much higher level than normal. This is done by energizing the muscles with Qi through the concentrated, meditative mind.

Although Xingyiquan is classified as an internal style, its theory and principles of defense and applications are different from those of the best-known internal style, Taijiquan. While Taijiquan emphasizes power that is as soft as a whip, Xingyiquan uses power which is like rattan—soft at the beginning and hard at the instant of striking. While Taijiquan emphasizes using defense as an offense, Xingyiquan emphasizes using offense as the defense. While Taijiquan focuses on middle and short range fighting techniques, Xingyiquan concentrates on short range fighting. In this, Xingyiquan's Jin (martial power, 勁) seems to resemble White Crane's, yet it has its own unique theories of defense and offense. Xingyiquan's power must always remain soft internally, yet it must be hard externally whenever necessary.

Although Xingyiquan has only five basic movements, their variations and applications are unlimited. It is like dancing the waltz—which has only three basic steps, but hundreds of variations. Therefore, although the beginner will find Xingyiquan easier to learn than many other arts, it will still take more than ten years of pondering and practice to reach the deeper level of understanding and application. Because of this, it is a good style for a beginner who does not have any experience in the internal styles. It is also good as a second internal style for those who have already learned one, and it will increase their understanding of their first style. For those who are only interested in health, Xingyiquan provides a few simple movements which will achieve that goal.

When you read this book, it is especially important for you to understand Xingyiquan's theories and principles. They will serve as a map, and provide you with clear directions to lead you to your goal in the shortest possible time. If you do not understand the theory, what you learn will be only flowers and branches, and it will have no root.

Preface—First Edition

Master Liang, Shou-Yu 梁守渝先生

When I was six years old, I started to train Qigong (氣功), which is related to Chinese martial arts. When I was eight, I began to learn and practice traditional Chinese Gongfu (功夫). Although I have been involved in teaching Wushu (武術) and Taiji Qigong (太極氣功) for more than twenty-five years, I have never written a martial arts book in a language other than Chinese. I have hesitated to write anything because, compared with the vast and profound domain of Chinese martial knowledge, my own understanding is so limited and unrefined. In addition to this, the political situation in mainland China has been so unsteady that writing has become one of the most difficult things to do there.

Since I arrived in North America in 1981, I have dedicated my best efforts to introducing the various marvelous forms of traditional Chinese Wushu to Western society. Although I had written a few Chinese books about martial arts training and a few articles related to the Emei style (峨嵋派) of martial arts, I have always felt that my English was not good enough to write a book in English.

In 1985 I had a chance to become acquainted with Dr. Yang, Jwing-Ming, and in no time we became the closest of friends. I really admire his talent both in scholarship and the martial arts. I respect him more highly for his sincerity, humility, and eagerness to help others. I also especially admire his morality in respecting teachers and elders, and the fact that he takes the real "Dao" (道) so seriously. In addition to teaching his students Wugong (武功)(martial Gongfu), he is also very serious about teaching them about martial morality and individual moral cultivation. This is an extremely precious virtue, especially in today's martial society. Because he is humble in treating others and in learning, he has gained many aspects of knowledge. Because of his intelligent study from books, his martial arts knowledge is abundant and vast. Everytime we meet, it is always the most joyful and happiest time for us. We learn from each other, we study and discuss. I feel I have really gained a lot of benefit from this.

The publication of this Xingyiquan book, as a matter of fact, is all Jwing-Ming's effort. What I have done is only introduce the movements and the sequences which I have learned. Because of this my name is listed as one of the authors. Therefore, for the publication of this book I would like to thank my brother, Dr. Yang, Jwing-Ming. I am also grateful to the others who have helped in completing this book.

Even though Dr. Yang and I have tried our best in this book to introduce the Xingyiquan arts to the Western world, the domain of Xingyiquan is so wide and its contents are so abundant and profound that there are still many voids which need to be filled. We sincerely wish that talented Xingyiquan masters will not hesitate to share their knowledge either through writing or through seminars with the public. In this way, through all of our efforts we will be able to promote the Chinese internal arts. Naturally, their suggestions on this book are quite welcome and appreciated.

Master Liang, Shou-Yu

Preface—First Edition

Dr. Yang, Jwing-Ming 楊俊敏博士

Although I have practiced Taijiquan (太極拳) for more than 27 years, it was not until the last few years that I realized that I have just started to taste the essence and comprehend the deep theory of the internal arts. I now consider myself to be only a beginner in the Chinese internal arts. This understanding has increased my desire to explore other internal martial styles such as Xingyiquan (形意拳) and Baguazhang (八卦掌), which have different theory from that of Taijiquan. However, because of my busy schedule and also because of the difficulty in finding a qualified teacher in the USA, I have never had the chance to explore another internal martial art.

It was not until 1985 that I was fortunate enough to meet Master Liang, Shou-Yu in Houston. I learned that he is a living repository of China's vest culture heritage in the field of internal and external martial arts and Qigong. We know that the emergence of a great master does not occur by mere coincidence of events. However, Master Liang did have all the advantages of being born into a martial arts family and having the chance to come into contact with many legendary grandmasters. Because of his love and utter devotion to the martial arts, and because of his characteristic perseverance and insight, Master Liang has made himself a superbly seasoned artist, striving for nothing less than the utmost precision and perfection of the art.

When we met and realized we both shared a love for the Chinese martial arts, we felt a sense of respect for each other. This soon grew into a feeling of brotherhood, and since then we have shared our knowledge openly, without doubt or hesitation.

When I found that Mr. Liang is also an expert in Xingyiquan, I asked him to teach me and my students. During this learning and teaching period, we felt that it would be a good idea to write a Xingyiquan book together. We felt that with my experience in writing and publishing, as well as my background in the internal arts and Qigong, and also with the assistance of many Xingyiquan books which were published earlier in this century, we should be able to write a systematic, theoretical analysis of the art. Since theory is the root and the foundation of any training, we believe that a theoretical discussion of Xingyiquan is necessary to help the practitioner increase his understanding and advance his training. Furthermore, in order to write a good book, I must dig into it deeply until I really understand it. This helps me to lay out the right path for my training.

Although I have been responsible for writing the theoretical portion, it has all been carefully checked by Master Liang. Since the forms and the postures are very important for teaching those who intend to learn from the book, they are demonstrated primarily by Master Liang himself. We hope that our mutual effort has resulted in a worthwhile book.

In this book, the first chapter will define Xingyiquan and explains its training content, survey its history, and review the life of its creator, Marshal Yue, Fei (岳飛). The second chapter will consist of a theoretical analysis of Xingyiquan, which will be based on the documents which have been passed down from ancient times in the form of poetry or songs. These documents will be first translated and then commented upon. This discussion will lead you into a deep theoretical understanding of Xingyiquan.

Since Xingyiquan is an internal martial art, it has routine forms for training the internal Qi. This is very common in almost all of the Chinese martial styles. In the third chapter, we will introduce the traditional Xingyiquan Qigong training. Through this training, not only will your health be significantly improved, but also your internal strength will be greatly increased. Chapter 4 will introduce the five most basic Xingyiquan movements. These five movements are the foundation of the entire art, and all the various techniques are derived from them. Only when you understand these five fundamental movements will you be able to understand the relationship between them of mutual production and conquest.

Once you understand the relationship of the five fundamental movements, you will be ready for the practice sequence in Chapter 5 which utilizes these movements. To help you go deeper into the art, Chapter 6 teaches an intermediate sequence. To help you understand the application of the Xingyiquan techniques, a two-men fighting set will be introduced in the seventh chapter. This will be followed with a conclusion in Chapter 8.

Readers who are interested in digging more into Xingyiquan theory should seriously study Appendix A. It contains the ten important training theses written by Marshal Yue, Fei, along with translation and commentary. These theses are the roots of the entire Xingyiquan training, and will lead you to a deep level of understanding.

Dr. Yang, Jwing-Ming

Preface—Second Edition

Dr. Yang, Jwing-Ming 楊俊敏博士

Since the first edition of this book was introduced to Chinese martial arts society in the West more than ten years ago, numerous interested western martial artists finally have had a better idea about this style of internal Chinese martial arts. Due to the limited number of qualified Xingyiquan instructors available, this internal art is not yet widespread and commonly practiced, it has served its main purpose. This purpose is to introduce another internal martial style that has a profound theoretic and philosophical foundation which was established from accumulation of Chinese historical experience and culture. We should understand that, though the development and the practice derived from this theory and philosophy can be many and different, its theoretical foundation and the spirit of the art remain the same. The most important aspect of this art is that through understanding this internal art, you will have another perspective to see a different level and horizon of the Chinese internal martial arts.

Xingyiquan was created by Marshal Yue, Fei (岳飛) nearly one thousand years ago. It was created as an army martial training so a new soldier had an opportunity to learn an effective martial art which allowed him to reach to a defensive and offensive capability in a short time. Therefore, there are only five basic martial strategic moving patterns. Though they are only five basic fighting patterns, its theory is profound and skills of fighting is extremely high. Since it was created as an army martial style, it emphases offense more than defense and straight forward more than backward. However, the most important part of the training is the spirit of the fighting. From this fighting spirit, a practitioner is able to bring his alertness, awareness, and fighting morale to a high level. All of these special and unique characteristics of this style can be seen in Marshal Yue's ten important thesis which are included in the Appendix of this book.

For the last ten years, many western internal martial artists, through reading and understanding the theory and the basic training patterns introduced from this book and videotapes, are able to pick up a correct feeling and practice in this art. This has led them to a correct path of another domain of internal arts. Since the entire human race has been gradually entering the new century—the century of spiritual development, this spiritual arts has become more important for those who wish to develop his spiritual development through martial arts training. Due to this reason, it is about the time to re-introduce this book to the readers.

The main differences of this new edition from the old one are: 1. All of the Chinese spelling has been changed into more popular Pinyin system; 2. All Chinese have been attached in the text for those who understand Chinese; 3. Some old errors have been corrected; and 4. Introduce some new concepts which have been understood by me in the last ten years. I hope through this new introduction of this book, Xingyiquan will become popular and thus benefit to those who are interested in Chinese martial arts and spiritual study.

Dr. Yang, Jwing-Ming

Acknowledgments

Thanks to A. Reza Farman-Farmaian for the photography, Wen-Ching Wu and Peter Dinh for describing the movements of the sequences, Tim Comrie for typesetting, and John R. Redmond for the cover drawing. Thanks also to Ramel Rones and Sam Masich for general help, to David Ripianzi, Jeffrey Pratt, Aaron Dumas and many other YMAA members for proofing the manuscript and for contributing many valuable suggestions and discussions. Special thanks to Alan Dougall for his editing.

General Introduction

一般介紹

1.1 INTRODUCTION

Although the internal styles of Chinese martial arts are becoming more popular in the Western world, many people still have questions about them. The most common questions are: what are the major differences between the external and internal martial styles? How is Qi related to these different styles? What are the differences between martial and non-martial Qigong? What are the differences in both theory and techniques between the different internal styles? You need to have the answers to these general questions before you can have an understanding of the role that Xingyiquan plays among the Chinese internal arts. Then you will be able to ask yourself why you want to learn Xingyiquan rather than Taijiquan or some other internal styles.

In this section, we will briefly answer all of these questions. To answer them fully would actually require a rather large book. It is almost like trying to describe the different tastes of various Chinese foods. You can get a general idea, but unless you actually sample them, you will not really understand what you are reading about. This is especially true in the Chinese internal arts, where the spiritual feeling and enlightenment are the ultimate goals.

1.1.1 Differences between the Internal and External Styles

Before we go into the differences between the internal and external styles, you should first recognize one important point: all of the Chinese styles, both internal and external, came from the same root. If a style does not share this root, then it is not a Chinese martial style. This root is the Chinese culture. Throughout the world, various races have created many different arts, each one based on that race's cultural background. Therefore, it does not matter which style you are discussing, as long as it was created in China, it must contain the essence of Chinese art, the spirit of traditional Chinese virtue, and the knowledge of traditional fighting techniques which have been passed down for thousands of years.

Martial artists of old looked at their experiences and realized that in a fight there are three factors which actually decided victory. These three factors are speed, power, and technique. Generally speaking, speed is the most important among the three. This is simply because, if you are fast, you can get to the opponent's vital areas more easily. Even if your power is weak and you only know a limited number of techniques, you still have a good chance of inflicting a serious injury on the opponent.

If you already have speed, then what you need is power. Even if you have good speed and techniques, if you don't have power your attacks and defense will not be as effective as they could be. You may have met people who had great muscular strength but no martial arts training who were able to defeat skilled martial artists who didn't have power. Finally, when you have good speed and power and if you can develop good techniques and a wise strategy, then there is no doubt that victory will belong to you. Therefore, in the Chinese martial arts, more than the study of techniques, increasing speed and improving power are the most important subjects.

It does not matter what techniques a style creates, they must all follow certain basic principles and rules. For example, all offensive and defensive techniques must effectively protect vital areas such as the eyes, throat, and groin. Naturally, when you attack, you must be able to access your opponent's vital areas without exposing your own.

It is the same with speed and power training. Although each style tried to keep their methods secret, they all followed the same general rules. For example, developing muscle power should not be detrimental to your speed, and developing speed should not decrease your muscular power. Both must be of equal concern. Furthermore, the training methods you use or develop should be appropriate to the techniques which are characteristic of your style. For example, in eagle and crane styles, the speed and power of the grabbing are extremely important and should be emphasized.

According to the available documents, before the Liang Dynasty (502-557 A.D., 梁朝) martial artists did not study how to use Qi to increase speed and power. After the Liang Dynasty martial artists realized the value of Qi training in developing speed and power, and it became one of the major concerns in almost all styles. Because of this, we should discuss this subject by dividing it into two eras. The dividing point should be the Liang Dynasty, when Da Mo (達磨) was preaching in China.

Before Da Mo, even though Qi theory and principles had been studied and widely applied in Chinese medicine, they were not used in the martial arts. Speed and power were generally developed through continued training. Even though the training emphasized a concentrated mind, they did not take the next step and link this to developing Qi. Instead, they concentrated solely on muscular power. For this reason, these styles are classified as external styles.

Then, the emperor Liang Wu (梁武帝) invited the Indian monk Da Mo to China to preach Buddhism. When the emperor did not agree with Da Mo's Buddhist philosophy, the monk went across the Yellow River (黃河) to the Shaolin Temple (少林寺). He saw that many priests were weak and fell asleep during his lectures. He decided to go into meditation to discover how to help the monks. After nine years of meditation in a cave, he wrote two classics, *Yi Jin Jing (Muscle/Tendon Changing Classic,* 易筋經) and *Xi Sui Jing (Marrow/Brain Washing Classic,* 洗髓經). After Da Mo died, the Shaolin priests continued to practice his methods, especially the Yi Jin Jing, to strengthen their bodies and spirits. They soon found that the training not only made them healthier, it also made them stronger. At that time, even priests needed to know martial arts to protect themselves from bandits. When they combined the Qi training with their traditional defense techniques they became very effective fighters. As Da Mo's training methods spread out from the Shaolin Temple, many forms of martial Qigong were developed. This is discussed more thoroughly in the book: *Qigong—The Secret of Youth* by Dr. Yang.

The Yi Jin Jing was not originally intended to be used for fighting. However, the martial Qigong based on it was able to significantly increase power, so it became a necessary training course in the Shaolin Temple. This had a revolutionary effect on Chinese martial arts, leading them to establish an internal foundation based on Qi training.

A short time after Da Mo died, several martial styles were created which emphasized a soft body, instead of the stiff muscular body developed by the Shaolin priests. The reasons for this were very simple. They believed that since Qi (internal energy, 氣) is the root and foundation of physical strength, a martial artist should first build up this internal root. When his Qi was abundant and full, it could energize the physical body to a higher level so that power could be manifested more effectively and efficiently. In order to build up the Qi and circulate it smoothly in the body, the body must be relaxed and the mind must be concentrated. We know of at least two internal styles which were created during this time (550-600 A.D.): Hou Tian Fa (Post Heaven Techniques, 後天法) and Xiao Jiu Tian (Small Nine Heavens, 小九天). According to some documents, these two styles were the original sources of Taijiquan, the creation of which is credited to Zhang, San-Feng (張三豐) of the late Song Dynasty (宋朝)(around 1200 A.D.).[1]

The various martial arts are divided into external and internal styles. While the external styles emphasize training techniques and building up the physical body through some martial Qigong training, the internal styles emphasize the build up of Qi in the body. In fact, all styles, both internal and external, have martial Qigong training. The external styles train the physical body and hard Qigong first, and gradually become soft and train soft Qigong; while the internal styles train soft Qigong first, and later apply the Qi built up to the physical techniques. It is said that: "The external styles are from hard to soft and the internal styles are from soft to hard, the ways are different but the final goal is the same."[2] It is also said: "External styles are from external to internal, while internal styles are from internal to external. Though the approaches are different, the final goal is the same."[3] Again, it is said: "External styles first Li (muscular strength) and then Qi, while internal styles first Qi and later Li."[4]

The preceding discussion should have given you a rough idea of how to distinguish external and internal styles. Frequently, internal and external styles are also judged by how the Jin (勁) is manifested. Jin is defined as "Li (力) and Qi (氣)," (Li means muscular strength). It is how the muscles are energized by the Qi and how this manifests externally as power. It is said: "the internal styles are as soft as a whip, the soft-hard styles (half external and half internal) are like rattan, and the external styles are like a staff." If you are interested in this rather large subject, please refer to Dr. Yang's books *Tai Chi Theory and Martial Power* and *The Essence of Shaolin White Crane*.

1.1.2 Qi, Health, and Martial Arts

First let us define Qi. The original meaning of the Chinese word Qi was "universal energy." Every type of energy in this universe is called Qi. When this term was later applied to the human body, it meant the energy which is maintained or circulated in the body. In the last twenty years, a clearer definition of the Qi which is circulating in the human body has arisen: bioelectric energy. All other types of energy in different forms, such as heat or light, are considered to be only transformation of bioelectric energy.

In this universe, Qi is the original energy source which keeps the entire universe alive. It is the same in the human body, where Qi keeps the various cells alive and keeps the physical body functioning. Your body is like an electric fan which needs electricity to make it turn. If the electric circulation is insufficient, the fan will not work properly. In the same way, if the Qi supply in your body is insufficient or stagnant, you will become sick or even die.

In Chinese Qigong, Qi is classified as Yin because it can only be felt, while the physical body is classified as Yang because it can be seen. Yin (陰) is the root and source of the life which animates the Yang (陽) body (physical body) and manifest power or strength externally. Therefore, when the Qi is strong, the physical body can function properly and be healthy, and it can manifest a lot of power or strength.

In order to have a healthy and strong body, you must learn how to keep the Qi circulating in your body smoothly, and you must also learn how to build up an abundant store of Qi. In order to reach these two goals, you must first understand the Qi circulatory and storage system in your body.

In your body, there are "twelve primary Qi channels" (十二經) which function like rivers and distribute Qi throughout your body. There are also eight "extraordinary Qi vessels" (八脈) which function like reservoirs, storing and regulating Qi in your body. One end of each channel is connected to one of the twelve internal

Laogong (P-8)

Figure 1-1. Laogong cavity

Yongquan (K-1)

Figure 1-2. Yongquan cavity

organs, while the other end is connected to either a finger or toe. These twelve Qi channels lead Qi to the twelve organs to nourish them and to keep them functioning properly. Whenever the Qi level circulating in the channels is abnormal due to stagnation or sickness, one or several organs will not receive the proper amount of Qi nourishment and will tend to malfunction.

The eight vessels include four in the body and four in the legs. These vessels store Qi, and are able to regulate the Qi flow in the twelve Qi channels. In addition, there are five gates through which the Qi in the body communicates with the Qi in the surrounding environment, and further help to regulate the body. The main gate is the head. There are four secondary gates: a Laogong (P-8)(勞宮) cavity in the center of each palm (Figure 1-1), and a Yongquan (K-1)(湧泉) cavity on the bottom of each foot (Figure 1-2). The tips of the fingers and toes are also considered lesser gates and help with the regulation of Qi. Furthermore, there are thousands of pores over the whole of your body which are also considered small gates which constantly regulate the body's Qi and therefore adjust the body's Yin and Yang.

In order to have a healthy body and slow down the aging process, you must learn how to keep the Qi circulating in the twelve channels smoothly, and you must learn how to fill up the Qi reservoirs so that they can regulate the Qi flow efficiently. You must also learn how the Qi in your body communicates with the Qi around you so that your body can adapt to natural conditions.

If you can understand Qi circulation theory in the human body, then you will be able to understand how Qi can be related to the martial arts. Remember that the human body is not a machine like the aforementioned electrical fan. It is alive, and able to improve itself. When your Qi grows stronger, your physical body will also grow stronger. Therefore, if you build your Qi up to a stronger level, your organs and physical body will receive more nourishment and their condition will improve, and you will also become stronger.

To make this clearer, remember that many parts of your body, such as the limbs, are governed by your mind. The governing process is very simple. Your mind generates an idea, and this thought leads Qi to the appropriate muscles to energize them so that they will perform the desired action. The key to martial Qigong training is learning how to lead your Qi more efficiently so that you can manifest more power. According to Western science, people normally never use their muscles at more than 40 to 50% of their maximum capability. This is simply because you don't need any more for your daily activities. This also implies that your mind has never been trained to lead the Qi more efficiently.

The Chinese martial artist learns how to concentrate his mind through meditation or other training so that it can lead his Qi efficiently. This significantly increases his power and makes his techniques more effective. The martial artist also learns through meditation to use his Qi to raise his spirit and also his morality. Through correct training, the mind can reach a very calm and peaceful state. The real "Dao" (道) of Chinese martial arts aims for both spirit and skills. The correct way of training is to perfect oneself both in techniques and spirit, not to conquer others. Only then can you obtain the full benefits of good health and lead a meaningful life.

1.1.3 Popular Chinese Internal Martial Arts

Because all Chinese martial styles utilize some Qigong training, it is difficult to distinguish the external styles from the internal. Traditionally, almost all of the Chinese martial styles were taught in secret, and it was not until the last 100 years that these secrets were gradually exposed to the general public. There are many styles that are still taught secretly. Because of this conservatism, most people (including many Chinese martial artists) do not have enough information to distinguish the styles clearly. There are four generally known styles which emphasize Qi development more seriously than other styles, and are therefore considered internal. These four styles are Taijiquan, Xingyiquan, Baguazhang, and Liu He Ba Fa. We would like to briefly introduce the major differences between these four styles.

Before we discuss these differences, we would first like to point out the similarities among these four styles. First, they all concentrate on training the circulation of Qi and building it up to a higher level. Second, they all emphasize a calm and peaceful mind. And finally, all four styles are very effective in improving health.

1. Taijiquan 太極拳

A. In order for the Qi to move freely and smoothly in the physical body, the body must be relaxed from the skin to the bone marrow and the internal organs. In order to lead the Qi to any part of the body without stagnation, in addition to the body being relaxed, the movements must be as soft as a baby's.

B. When Jin (勁) is emitted for an attack, it is like a whip. Though soft, the power is strong and penetrating.

C. The fighting strategy is more defensive than offensive. This means that defense is often treated as the preparation for an attack. Because of this, training focuses on yielding, neutralizing, sticking, adhering, and coiling, and movements are always rounded. "Pushing hands" practice leads the practitioner to this goal.

D. Strategy and techniques indicate that Taijiquan specializes in fighting mostly in the short and middle ranges. Almost all of the kicks trained in the Taijiquan sequences focus within these ranges.

2. Xingyiquan 形意拳

A. In order to enable the Qi to move freely and smoothly in the physical body, the body must be natural and comfortable. In the beginning of both attacking and defensive movements, the body remains soft so that Qi can be led to the limbs. The body is then stiffened for an instant upon striking to manifest the Jin. Xingyi Jin is like rattan, soft at the beginning and hard at the end. Jin manifests like a cannonball exploding.

B. The fighting strategy is more active than passive. Offensive movement is usually used as a defense. Although techniques such as yielding, neutralizing, sticking, adhering, and coiling are used, the attacking mind and movement remain paramount. In order to keep up momentum, straight forward and backward movements are emphasized, although some dodging and sideward movements are used.

C. Because of the strategy and techniques emphasized, Xingyiquan can be very effective within the short fighting range. Though some kicks are trained, almost all of them are directed at targets below the groin.

3. Baguazhang 八卦掌

A. The movements of Baguazhang are not as soft as Taijiquan, yet they are not as hard as Xingyiquan. The internal Qi is the main focus of the training.

B. The fighting strategy emphasizes circular movements. Both the stepping and the techniques are circular. Although many techniques such as yielding, neutralizing, sticking, adhering, and coiling are used, they are mainly adopted to coordinate with the round movements. Attack and defense are equally important. Rounded defensive movements are usually used first, followed by rounded attacking movements to uproot the opponent and make him fall.

C. Because of its strategy and techniques, Baguazhang can be effective at all ranges. Because round stepping movements are constantly used in coordination with the techniques, kicks are seldom used. The training focuses instead on firm and rapid walking.

4. Liu He Ba Fa 六合八法

Liu He Ba Fa is a combination of the strategy and techniques of Taijiquan, Xingyiquan, and Baguazhang. Therefore, the training contains soft within the hard and hard within the soft. Its strategy contains straight line forward and backward, as well as circular movements. It utilizes all three fighting ranges. It does not emphasize kicking techniques. It is normally taught to people who have already learned the three styles, because they are most likely to be able to understand the essence of the three and mix the techniques skillfully and apply them effectively.

1.1.4 Why Learn Xingyiquan?

Each of the styles discussed above has its own characteristics and its own advantages. You may have decided that one of them may be better for you. The effectiveness of the techniques and strategy depend upon the actual situation and your opponent's expertise. If fact, very often you will find that one who spends a relatively short time learning and mastering an easier style is able to defeat an opponent who has practiced a more difficult style for a long time. Remember, learning a few useful things is better than learning a lot of things you cannot use. The best approach in learning anything is to master a few things and comprehend them deeply, rather than learning a lot and staying on the surface.

Next, we will summarize some advantages of learning Xingyiquan. Hopefully this will give you a clearer idea of whether or not you would like to learn this art.

1. The basic forms are simple and easy to learn. Xingyiquan is like the Waltz—there are only a few simple moves, so it is easy to learn. Like the Waltz, there are hundreds of variations derived from the basic movements, and their applications are countless. Therefore, it is very suitable for beginners who are interested in understanding the internal styles of Chinese martial arts. Also, because of its countless variations, after one has mastered the basic movements, Xingyiquan can be used as a second style for those who already have some experience in internal arts.

2. The fundamental theory and training principles are easy to understand. Therefore, it is very easy for a beginner to have a firm comprehension of the theory of the style right from the beginning. In most other systems you have to practice for many years before you comprehend the essence of the style. As your training progresses you will find that your understanding of the theory deepens in regard to both health and martial arts. Like Newton's equations, they look simple, but the derivations from the equations are deep and many. The depth of Xingyiquan theory makes it suitable for those experienced internal martial artists who would like to compare the essence of Xingyiquan with their original style. Remember the more angles you look at something from, the better you will understand it.

3. From the point of view of health, the movements of Xingyiquan are designed for strengthening the five important Yin organs: heart, lungs, kidneys, liver, and spleen. Practicing these five basic movements will remove stagnant Qi and smooth out the Qi circulation, and build up the health of the organs.

4. The theory of Xingyiquan's fighting strategy is based on the mutual relationships of production and conquest of the Five Phases (Wuxing, 五行). Through these relationships, the five basic movements can be skillfully combined to make a very effective fighting style. A style which is simple to learn and has simple fighting principles is often more effective than styles which have many complicated techniques and an involved fighting theory.

5. The deeper advantage of practicing Xingyiquan is probably in the spiritual realm. Xingyiquan's theory and techniques are aggressive, yet the practitioner avoids emotional excitement. Xingyiquan manifests great power, but it is a very refined power, and while the strategy is offensive, it is not disordered. Continued training in Xingyiquan can make you spiritually brave so that you will be able to face challenges with equanimity. Your spirit can be raised to a very powerful stage, yet you will remain calm, peaceful, and in control. This is essential for facing this world and leading a meaningful life. When you read the poetry and songs in the second chapter, try to catch the spiritual feeling and understand the profound meaning of the style.

1.2 WHAT IS XINGYIQUAN?

In order to survive in what is oftentimes a violent and cruel world, animals must very quickly develop the ability to protect themselves from natural dangers and other animals. All wild animals still have the instincts and senses for this. They all still know how to hunt and fight to survive. These abilities require physical strength, a natural, instinctively perceptive mind, and a highly alert spirit. For example, an eagle must have sharp eyes and claws. A tiger doesn't just need a strong body and claws, it must also have the spirit which makes other animals afraid of it.

We humans have lost most of the natural instincts, senses, and fighting abilities that all other animals possess. In order to regain these abilities and use them to fight against other men, the martial artists in ancient times imitated the fighting techniques and spirits of animals, modifying them with human rational analysis. This is how many different styles were created.

Xingyiquan was created in imitation of the fighting techniques and spirit of twelve animals. One of the documents which are available to us contains a section which explains what Xingyiquan is. We would like to translate it here and make some comments. Hopefully this will give you a clear concept of Xingyiquan.

About Xingyi 形意說

(What is) the Xing (the shape)? The shape of imitating. (What is) the Yi (the mind)? The mind (generated) from the Xin (heart).

形者，形象也。意者，心意也。

"Shape" (Xing, 形) here means the external appearance or the movements used in fighting, and Yi (意)(pronounce ee) means the mind which is generated internally from the heart (Xin, the emotional, feeling mind)(心). Therefore, Xingyiquan is an internal style which imitates the shapes of twelve animals and their inner characteristics when they fight.

According to Chinese Qigong, Yi (意) is the wisdom mind, which is generated from the Xin (心)(emotional mind). The emotional mind makes you excited, quick, and agile, while the wisdom mind makes you calm and gives you clear and accurate judgement. When you are able to combine your Xin and Yi, your movements will be fast and agile, yet accurate and calm.

Therefore, Xingyiquan is an internal martial art which utilizes the techniques of the twelve animals, and also requires an internal cultivation by which the Xin and Yi can be combined.

(Only) man of the million living things has a "Ling" (supernatural spirit). (He) is able to feel and respond to everything. This is because (he has a) Xin (emotional mind) internally to comprehend the surrounding objects. Objects are external, but the "comprehending" is internal.

人為萬物之靈，能感通諸事之應，是以心在內，而理周乎物，物在外，而理具於心。

"Ling" (靈) means supernatural spirit. The Chinese people believe that men are more civilized and wiser than other animals simply because they have a "Ling" which allows them to feel, understand, and communicate with nature. All of this is because we have stronger emotional feelings than other animals. The outside of your body and everything external to you is comprehended by your mind, which is within you. The control of your body's posture and movement also comes from your internal awareness and understanding.

The Yi (wise judgement) originates with the Xin (emotional mind). Therefore, (when) Xin and Yi sincerely exist within, then millions of objects will be shaped externally. The internal and external correspondence (depends on) nothing but the circulation and transport of the one Qi.

意者，心之所發也；是故心意成於中，而萬事形於外，內外相感，不外一氣之流行。

Your Yi (wisdom mind) originates with your Xin (heart, or emotional mind). This is because it is your emotional mind which first responds to stimuli. Your wisdom mind evaluates what the emotional mind has perceived. If your wisdom mind is in control of your emotional mind, and they both sincerely work together, then you will have great control of everything external, both your body's posture and movements, and your interactions with people and things around you ("millions of objects"). This control is the result of having strong, healthy Qi circulation, and also of being able to effectively move the Qi wherever you wish.

> *Therefore Da Mo, the ancestral teacher, used this (theory) and created this fist (i.e., style). His objective was Yang Qi (i.e., cultivating Qi) and increasing the Li (muscular strength). The movements are simple, but its achievements and applications are unlimited. Therefore, it is named Xingyi (Shape-Mind) Quan (Fist).*

> 故達磨祖師本之，而創是拳，其旨在養氣，在益力，動作簡而功用無窮，故名之曰〝形意拳〞也。

It is believed that Marshal Yue, Fei was the creator of Xingyiquan. However, since his art originated at Shaolin, many martial artists credit Da Mo as the original ancestor.

Many people think that Shaolin Gongfu is limited to the external techniques, but they are wrong. All of the Chinese martial styles require internal training to build up the Qi in order to reach a high level of skill. Xingyiquan is a typical example. It emphasizes Yang Qi (養氣). Yang (養) means to nourish, to increase, to raise, and to cultivate. Only after you have built up your Qi to a higher level will you be able to use it to effectively energize the muscles and increase your power. Muscle power is called "Li" (力). Li is the demonstration of muscular power, but it must be energized by Qi (refer to Dr. Yang's books: *Tai Chi Theory and Martial Power,* also *The Essence of Shaolin White Crane*).

1.3 HISTORY OF XINGYIQUAN

The history of the martial arts before the Qing Dynasty (1644 A.D.)(清朝) is very vague because almost all of the Chinese martial artists were conservative and the styles were passed down secretly. It is the same with Xingyiquan. According to most of the available documents, the origin of Xingyiquan should probably be dated at least as far back as the Liang Dynasty (502-557 A.D.)(梁朝) at the Shaolin Temple (少林寺). This is because, at this time, the Shaolin Temple was already imitating the movements and fighting spirit of five animals in their martial arts training. Later, during the Southern Song Dynasty (1127-1280 A.D.)(南宋), it is believed that Zhang, San-Feng (張三豐) combined the concepts of Shaolin martial arts with his own understanding of Qi and created Taijiquan. In fact, many Xingyiquan practitioners believed that Xingyiquan originated at Wudang Mountain (武當山), the same as Taijiquan did.

Since the late Southern Song Dynasty, when the soldiers in Marshal Yue's army were trained in Xingyiquan, the art has become very popular, and Marshal Yue is frequently credited with creating the art. However, since his martial arts originally came from the Shaolin Temple, many people trace Xingyiquan's ancestry back to the Shaolin Temple.

Between the Song and the late Ming Dynasties (宋、明), the history of Xingyiquan is again unclear. During the Qing Dynasty (1644-1912 A.D.), Xingyiquan became more popular because the mind of the Chinese people was more open, due in part to the more frequent contacts with Western culture. Consequently, its history during this period is better known.

Generally, it is believed that a martial artist named Ji, Ji-Ke (姬際可)(nicknamed Long-Feng)(隆豐) of Pu Zhou (浦州), who traveled and visited the well known masters in the mountains of Sichuan (四川省) and Shanxi Provinces (山西省), obtained on Zhong Nan Mountain (終南山) a secret book on Xingyiquan written by Marshal Yue. After he studied the art for some time, he passed it down to his disciple Cao, Ji-Wu (曹繼武), who in turn passed it down to Ji, Shou (姬壽) and Ma, Xue-Li (馬學禮). Ji, Shou later published Yue's book and popularized the art even more.

There have been many famous Xingyiquan masters since then. From then (Qing Tong Zhi, 清同治, 1862-1875 A.D.) until now, countless people have learned Xingyiquan. Here we can only name some of the best-known ones. There were Dai, Long-Bang (戴龍邦) and his brother Dai, Ling-Bang (戴陵邦) who learned from Ma, Xue-Li during the Qing Xian Feng period (清咸豐)(1851-1862 A.D.). Then they passed the art down to Li, Luo-Neng (李洛能). Li, Luo-Neng then passed it down to many of his students, the better-known ones being Song, Shi-Rong (宋世榮), Che, Yong-Hong (車永鴻), Liu, Qi-Lan (劉奇蘭), Guo, Yun-Shen (郭雲深), and Bo, Xi-Yuan (白西園). Among these five, Liu, Qi-Lan had many students such as his three sons, Liu, Jin-Tang (劉錦堂), Liu, Dian-Chen (劉殿琛), Liu, Rong-Tang (劉榮堂), and students Li, Cun-Yi (李存義), Zhou, Ming-Tai (周明泰), Zhang, Zhan-Kui (張占魁), Zhao, Zhen-Biao (趙振標), and Geng, Ji-Shan (耿繼善). Also, Guo, Yun-Shen passed down his arts to Liu, Yong-Qi (劉勇奇), Li, Kui-Yuan (李魁元), and Qian, Yan-Tang (錢硯堂).

In the beginning of this century, when the Qing emperor fell and the republic was organized by Dr. Sun, Yat-Sen (孫逸仙), the entire country entered a new era. As the nation gradually became more open-minded, the traditional secrets were more easily revealed to the public, and an enormous number of people took up Xingyiquan. For example, Li, Cun-Yi and Zhang, Zhan-Kui had a great many students, among them Li, Yun-Shan (李雲山) and Shang, Yun-Xiang (尚雲祥). Shang, Yun-Xiang's student Jin, Yun-Ting (靳雲亭) was a well known Xingyiquan promoter fifty years ago. Also, Li, Kui-Yuan's student Sun, Lu-Tang (孫祿堂) was well-known as a Taijiquan, Xingyiquan, and Baguazhang master. Finally, Zheng, Huai-Xian (鄭懷賢) learned from Sun, Lu-Tang and passed his arts to master Liang, Shou-Yu (梁守渝).

You can see that a chart of the generations of Xingyiquan masters would be very complicated. Keep in mind, also, that there are probably at least ten times as many people who also reached a high level of mastery, but are not well-known because they did not share their knowledge so generously with the public. This implies that the people mentioned were not necessarily the best Xingyiquan players of their time. (A similar thing happened with Taijiquan. A great many people throughout the world know about Yang, Cheng-Fu (楊澄甫) and his style of Taijiquan, but fewer people know about his uncles and the generation older than his uncles whose techniques were said to be much higher than his.)

Because the origin of Xingyiquan is so unclear, many martial artists would therefore credit Marshal Yue, Fei with its creation. There are several reasons for this. First, Marshal Yue, Fei was a Chinese hero and is respected by all Chinese. Second, Yue, Fei's martial arts came from the Shaolin Temple, which is considered the origin of both the internal and external styles. Third, Yue, Fei's ten theses on Xingyiquan demonstrate a very deep understanding of the art. Even though he may not be the creator, his theses have shown us the correct way to master the art. Fourth, Yue, Fei compiled and organized the Xingyiquan style into an effective martial system to train his soldiers. He is believed to be the first person to reveal the secrets of Xingyiquan to the public. Fifth, Yue, Fei was not only an expert in martial arts, he was also well known as a Qigong master. He is credited with creating the Eight Pieces of Brocade (Ba Duan Jin, 八段錦), which is a medical Qigong set for health, and the external martial style Yue Jia Ying Zhua (岳家鷹爪) (Yue Family's Eagle Claw). It is believed that only a person who was an expert in both Chinese medicine and martial arts would be able to combine them to create these styles.

Because of these reasons, and because almost all of the theory and principles discussed in this book are based on Yue, Fei theses, we would like to give you a brief biographical sketch of Marshal Yue, Fei.

1.4 Marshal Yue, Fei

The Song Dynasty (宋朝) (960-1280 A.D.) in China was a sorrowful time for the Chinese. Wars with the northern barbarians (the Jin race or Mongolian)(金人), corruption in business and government, and the specter of starvation constantly oppressed the people. But in the midst of all these troubles there arose a man who showed by the purity of his spirit and ideals that goodness, righteousness, and loyalty were qualities that still lived. For countless generations after his betrayal and murder at the hands of traitors, Marshal Yue, Fei (Figure 1-3) remains the ideal for the Chinese people of the completely virtuous man. In peace Yue, Fei was a great scholar of the Chinese classics, in war Yue, Fei was a brave and shrewd general who skill-

Figure 1-3. Marshal Yue, Fei and a sample of his calligraphy

fully defeated the enemies of his country.

Yue, Fei was born on February 15th, 1103 A.D. in Tang Yin Xian, Henan Province (河南、湯陰縣). While he was being born, a momentous event took place: a large, powerful bird called a Peng (鵬) flew onto the roof and began to make a tremendous noise. The father sensed that the bird's presence was an omen which foretold a tumultuous yet inspired fate for his son; the father thus named his son Fei (飛) which in Chinese means "to fly." This reflected the father's belief that his son would fly to great and noble heights as a man.

When Yue, Fei was but one month old, tragedy struck: the Yellow River (黃河) flooded. Yue, Fei's mother saved herself and her infant son by taking refuge in a giant urn; the urn acted as a small boat and took both mother and son to safety. When they reached dry land and the flood had receded, they went back to find that their home and property had been totally destroyed.

Yue, Fei's mother was very poor, but she was a well-educated scholar, and possessed the courage, intelligence, and bravery to raise her son properly and give him noble ideals. Because they were too poor to pay for an education, Yue, Fei's mother taught him personally. Each day she taught him how to read and write by drawing figures in the sand. Even though he lacked the books, paper, and brushes that other children had, the poor Yue, Fei became one of the best educated youngsters in his village; few children could match his scholarship.

In many ways the most important person and the greatest influence on Yue, Fei's life was his mother. All the ideals that Yue, Fei lived and died for were taught to him by his mother as they held their own classes using the sand as a blackboard. Without his mother's teachings and example, Yue, Fei would never have become the brave, intelligent, and loyal leader that he was.

The young Yue, Fei was a very avid reader. His favorite subjects were history and military theory. The book he admired and studied the most was *Sun's Book of Tactics*

(*Sun Zi Bing Fa*, 孫子兵法) by Sun, Wu (c. 557 B.C.)(孫武), which described the theory and practice of warfare. From this book Yue learned important principles which later helped him in his military career.

When Yue, Fei was a young man he became a tenant farmer for a landlord named Han, Qi (韓琦). After long hours of work he would come home to continue studying with his mother. Yue, Fei was much admired for this, and for the great physical strength he showed as a young man. As in scholarship, no one could match his natural power and speed.

These admirable qualities were noticed by a certain man in the town called Zhou, Tong (周侗). Zhou, Tong himself was a scholar and a very good martial artist who had studied in the Shaolin Temple. Seeing that Yue, Fei possessed many noble qualities, Zhou, Tong began to teach him martial arts. Martial arts as it was taught to Yue, Fei was a complete system involving barehand combat, weapons, military tactics, horsemanship, archery, and other related subjects. By constant practice Yue, Fei mastered everything Zhou, Tong taught.

When Yue, Fei was nineteen years old (1122 A.D.) he decided to aid his country by joining the Song army in its war against the Jin, a nomadic people who had invaded the Northern Song. The Song Dynasty, which was originally located in northern China, had to move to the south to re-establish itself with a new capital and emperor because the Jin had sacked their old capital and captured their emperor. The Song Dynasty which was invaded is known as the Northern Song (北宋)(960-1127 A.D.), while the Song Dynasty that established itself in the South after the Jin invasion is known as the Southern Song (南宋)(1127-1280 A.D.). For years the weakened Southern Song had to pay tribute to the Jin to keep them from attacking further south. When Yue, Fei joined the army, the Southern Song was trying to regain its lost land by war.

Yue, Fei proved himself to be an extraordinary soldier. His wisdom, bravery, and martial skill earned him promotion after promotion so that he became a general after only six years. Later, Yue, Fei became the commander or marshal of the army that was assigned to fight the Jin. Upon assuming command, he instituted a systematic training program in martial arts for his soldiers. Although some martial training had previously existed, Yue, Fei was the first to introduce Wushu (武術) into the army as a basic requirement before combat. Many times a young man joined the army only to find himself in battle the very next day. After a while, Yue's troops, known as Yue Jia Jun (岳家軍)(Yue Family Troop) became a highly efficient and successful fighting unit.

The success of Yue's troops can be basically attributed to three things. First, he made all his training strict; the troops were trained in a serious and professional manner. The soldiers were pushed until they excelled in martial arts. Second, Yue, Fei set up a military organization that was efficient and well run. Third, and most important, Yue, Fei created for his troops two new styles of Wushu. The first style which he taught to the troops came from his internal training, and led to the creation of Xingyiquan. The second style, which he created out of external Wushu, was Eagle Claw (鷹爪), a style which put a major emphasis on Qin Na (擒拿). The external style, because it was learned more easily, and because it had immediately practical techniques, made Yue's troops successful in battle.

With his highly trained troops Yue, Fei was in favor of pressing the attack against the Jin. He was so loyal and patriotic that he felt it was shameful for the Song to pay the Jin tribute. Yue, Fei constantly felt intense personal agony from the humiliation that his country suffered. With the desire to free his country constantly on his mind, Yue, Fei on his own initiative advanced his troops against the Jin to win back honor for the Song.

When Yue, Fei went into battle, his highly trained troops had many victories as they began to march north. But Yue, Fei had not yet encountered the Jin commander Wu Zhu (兀朮), who himself had never lost a battle. Wu Zhu's terrifying success was largely due to his main weapon—the feared Guai Zi Ma (拐子馬). The Guai Zi Ma was an ancient version of the tank. It was a chariot carrying armored men, drawn by three fully armored horses which were connected by a chain. It was extremely difficult to disable either the horses or the riders, and so they completely dominated the battlefield.

Yue, Fei had given much thought to defending against the awful Guai Zi Ma. As in other cases, Yue's brilliant military mind came up with a solution. He found that the horses were not protected in one place—their legs; putting armor on the horses' legs would have made them immobile. It was too difficult to attack the horses' legs with conventional arrows and spears, so Yue, Fei devised two simple but effective weapons: a sword with a hooked end, which was extremely sharp on the inside edge of the hook, and a shield made out of a vine called "rattan" (Teng, 藤). This army was called Teng Pai Jun (藤牌軍), or "The Rattan Shield Army."

At last, both generals met on a fateful day. When the battle started, Yue, Fei had the Rattan Shield Army crouching very low in the path of the Guai Zi Ma. Before the chariots could reach the soldiers, they ran into obstacles such as ditches and upright spears which Yue, Fei had had set up. Once these slowed down the chariots, Yue, Fei's soldiers, who were mainly on foot, could move against the enemy with more ease. As the chariots advanced, the crouching men hooked and cut the legs of the horses, making them fall. It was impossible for the horses to trample the crouching men because the shields were greased, and the horses slipped every time they put their feet on them. When the crouching soldiers attacked the horses they only had to cripple one animal to stop a chariot. Once a chariot was stopped, other soldiers surrounded it and killed the riders. On that day Yue, Fei scored a military victory which lives today in history and legend.

Yue, Fei then proceeded north, regaining lost territory and defeating such Jin generals as the Tiger King and Great Dragon. But while Yue, Fei was regaining his country's honor, the Jin leaders successfully bribed one of the most infamous men in Chinese history—Qin, Kuai (秦檜) to stop Yue, Fei. Qin, Kuai was at that time the prime minister, and the most influential man at the emperor's corrupt court.

While Yue, Fei's army moved north, Qin, Kuai, to accomplish his evil act, decided to send an imperial order with the emperor's official golden seal (Jin Pai, 金牌), asking Yue, Fei to come back. According to tradition, a general fighting on the front line had the option of refusing an order to retreat. Qin, Kuai was counting on Yue, Fei's patriotic sense of loyalty to the emperor to get him back. To ensure Yue, Fei's return Qin, Kuai sent twelve gold-sealed orders in one day; so much pressure made Yue, Fei return.

When Yue, Fei returned he was immediately imprisoned. Because Qin, Kuai feared that any sort of trial would reveal Yue, Fei's innocence, he ordered an officer named He, Zhu (何鑄) to thoroughly investigate Yue, Fei's life in an attempt to find some excuse for the imprisonment. He, Zhu searched and searched, but he found nothing. Although a powerful general, Yue, Fei had never abused his position for bad purposes. He, Zhu found that Yue, Fei had lived a spartan life, and had fewer possessions than a peasant. When He, Zhu returned to Qin, Kuai, he reported only one fact of significance. When Yue, Fei joined the army his mother tattooed on his back a certain phrase: "be loyal and pure to serve your country" (Jing Zhong Bao Guo, 精忠報國).

With such an honest general as Yue, Fei, Qin, Kuai had only one alternative—to have his food poisoned. Thus was the noble general viciously betrayed by his own countrymen. Without the glory and honor that was his right, Yue, Fei died in jail on January 27, 1142 A.D. (December 29, 1141 A.D. Chinese calendar). Yue, Fei was thirty-eight years old. Later, Yue, Fei's adopted son, Yue, Yun (岳雲), and Yue, Fei's top assistant, Zhang, Xian (張憲), were also killed.

For twenty years Yue, Fei was officially considered a criminal. But in 1166 A.D. a new and better government and emperor (Xiao Zong, 孝宗) took control. They refused to believe in the treachery of Yue, Fei, and relocated his grave to the beautiful West Lake (Xi Hu, 西湖) in Hangzhou (杭州). In front of the grave are stone statues of Qin, Kuai and his wife (Figure 1-4), kneeling in repentance and shame before Yue, Fei. These statues have to be replaced periodically, because many of the people who come to worship at the grave will deface or damage them out of anger at their treachery. Emperor Xiao Zong bestowed upon Yue, Fei a new name which symbolized what he always was and always will be: Yue Wu Mu (岳武穆) Yue, the righteous and respectable warrior."

1.5 THE CONTENTS OF XINGYIQUAN

It is important to know just what the art of Xingyiquan consists of, so that you will be able to evaluate where you stand in your training. It is said that the Xingyiquan passed down in the North by Li, Luo-Neng (李洛能) consisted of only the Five

Phases (Wu Xing, 五行) or Five Fists (Wu Quan, 五拳), the Linking Sequence (Lian Huan Quan, 連環拳), and the Twelve Shapes (Shi Er Xing, 十二形). Later Li's student Guo, Yun-Shen (郭雲深) and Gou's student Li, Cun-Yi (李存義) visited all of the well known Xingyiquan masters and compiled Xingyiquan into a more complete system.

Their new system consists of the Five Phases (or Five Fists), which include Pi (劈), Zuan (鑽), Beng (弸), Pao

Figure 1-4. Statues of Qin, Kuai and his wife

(炮), and Heng (橫), as the basic movements which correspond to the Five Phases in the *Yi Jing* (易經)(*Book of Changes*): Metal (Jin, 金), Water (Shui, 水), Wood (Mu, 木), Fire (Huo, 火), and Earth (Tu, 土). These five movements conform to the creation and conquest relationships of the Five Phases, which were used in the creation of the sequence named Five Phases Strike (Wu Xing Pao, 五行炮). This sequence was designed to help the student understand how to use the principles of mutual production and mutual conquest of the Five Phases.

Xingyiquan also includes a Five Phases Linking Sequence (Wu Xing Lian Huan Quan, 五行連環拳). This trains combining the Five Phases (五行)(or Five Fists, 五拳) and learning how to apply them in a continuous way based on the theory of the Five Phases. This sequence emphasizes threading the Qi into one.

There is also the Twelve Shapes (Shi Er Xing, 十二形) sequence which imitates the shapes and ways of fighting of twelve animals: Dragon (Long, 龍), Tiger (Hu, 虎), Snake (She, 蛇), Eagle (Ying, 鷹), Bear (Xiong, 熊), Monkey (Hou, 猴), Horse (Ma, 馬), Water Lizard (Tuo, 鼉), Chicken (Ji, 雞), Harrier (Yao, 鷂), Chinese Ostrich (Yi, 鴕), and Swallow (Yan, 燕). There is also a sequence named Miscellaneous Strikes (Za Shi Chui, 雜式捶), which is derived from the essence of the twelve shape sequence which threads the refined techniques into one.

In order to train a practitioner in the actual applications of the style, a matching set was created. It is called Secure Body Strike (An Shen Pao, 安身炮). The techniques of An Shen Pao are based on the pattern of the Five Phases (or Five Fists). This matching practice gives the beginner a grasp of the basic concept of how Xingyiquan works in an actual fight.

There are a few other sequences such as Eight Postures Sequence (Ba Shi Quan, 八式拳), Five Shape Saber (Wu Xing Dao, 五形刀), Five Shape Sword (Wu Xing Jian,

五形劍), Twelve Shape Spear (Shi Er Xing Qiang, 十二形槍), and Twelve Shape Staff (Shi Er Xing Gun, 十二形棍). However, only a few people today still preserve these rare forms. It is believed that learning these forms requires at least 10 years of training under a qualified instructor. Few students today can reach this level.

You can see that Xingyiquan is not like many other Chinese martial styles which may have fifty or even a hundred training sequences or routines. Like Taijiquan, the training sequences are few, but the essence is hidden deep and the knowledge and applications are profound.

References

1. "太極拳，刀、劍、桿、散手合編" (*Tai Chi Chuan: Saber, Sword, Staff, and Sparring*), Chen, Yan-Lin (陳炎林), Reprinted in Taipei, Taiwan, 1943.

2. 外家由硬而軟，內家由軟而硬，其法雖異，其的則同。

3. 外家由外而內，內家由內而外，其途雖異，其終的則一致。

4. 外家先力爾氣，內家先氣後力。

The Foundation of Xingyiquan 形意拳之基礎

2.1 INTRODUCTION

Like Taijiquan, but unlike external styles, Xingyiquan has only a limited number of practice routines which reflect the depth and profundity of the art's principles. This means that while it is easy to learn Xingyiquan, it is hard to comprehend the deeper essence and meaning of the art. Xingyiquan is considered an internal martial art, and it emphasizes nourishing Qi (Yang Qi, 養氣). It follows Qigong theory and training principles, which include converting essence into Qi (Lian Jing Hua Qi, 練精化氣), using the Qi to nourish the spirit (Lian Qi Hua Shen, 練氣化神), and finally purifying the spirit and learning the real meaning of the natural Dao (Lian Shen Fan Xu, 練神返虛).

Since Xingyiquan was created nearly one thousand years ago, many masters have written poems or songs about their experience of the essence of the art, and passed them down secretly through the generations. The reason they used poems and songs was simply that most Xingyiquan practitioners were illiterate. The pattern of the poetry would help the practitioners remember the key points until, after years of study and practice, they comprehended the essence of the art.

In this chapter we will include many of these poems and songs, translate them, and make some comments on them. Since historical records for this period are sporadic and unclear, it is difficult to learn the identities of the authors of these poems and songs. Our major sources for these documents are the Xingyiquan books published seventy-one years ago (1929 A.D.) by Ling, Gui-Qing (凌桂青)(*The Illustration of Xingyiquan*)[1] and by Jiang, Rong-Qiao (姜容樵)(*The Mother Fist of Xingyiquan*).[2] Most of these works were derived from Marshal Yue, Fei's original Xingyiquan theses, and explain the theory and fighting principles at a simpler level. Therefore, these works will be discussed in the main text of this book. Marshal Yue, Fei's ten important theses require a higher level of understanding, and so they will be translated and commented on in Appendix A. Once the reader understands the main text of this book, and has practiced for several years, he or she will then be able to use the study of Yue, Fei's work to deepen his level of understanding and feeling of the art.

When we translate these poems and songs, we will try as well as possible to retain the pattern and flavor which is expressed in the original Chinese. When necessary, extra words which are not in the original Chinese text will be added in parentheses to make the meaning clearer, or to smooth out the English and make it more idiomatic. Also, certain Chinese words which cannot be translated clearly into English are included in the text, followed by an approximate translation in parentheses. We hope that our efforts make it possible for you to grasp the real meaning and flavor of these documents.

Since most of these works are drawn from two major sources, many times you will discover that there are two different approaches to the same subject. We include both in the hope that this will help you to understand more easily.

2.2 The Foundation of Xingyiquan

Wuji Song 無極歌

Man is born in this grand space, no fighting and no competition. This place which the Yi can reach is complete, there is no blemish or shadow that can be found.

人生太空，無爭無競，意境渾然，不著蹤影。

Wuji (無極) means "no poles," and refers to the state where nothing is distinguished from anything else. In your personal life, Wuji is the state where you are not in conflict with people or within yourself. You are emotionally neutral because there are no forces pulling you away from your center. Then there is no trace or sign of your presence to disturb the harmony. When you are in this state your mind is clear and you can see things clearly. Since you are emotionally neutral, you can respond to events appropriately, without any interference from your emotions or preconceptions. If there is a need, you fill it, but it is almost as if you weren't there. Your wisdom mind (Yi, 意) alone controls your actions.

This song implies that one's mind should always be neutral and should not be disturbed by a sense of fighting, struggling, or competition. Only in this neutral state can your Yi reach a high stage of completeness. Completeness has the sense of being round and full, so that no force is able to destroy it, or even to judge, evaluate, or dissect it. In this case, there is no gap or defect which can be used to divide it.

In Xingyiquan, the beginning standing stance is called the Wuji posture (Wuji Shi, 無極式). Your mind stays at your center (Dan Tian, 丹田), and is calm and peaceful. Your body feels like a ball which is filling up with Qi, inflating evenly in all directions. Since your body and mind are centered and peaceful, there is nothing to upset or disturb you physically, mentally, or emotionally. No part of your posture sticks out unduly, or is unnecessarily withdrawn. There are no "extremes," and so you are in a Wuji state. The next song describes how your mind should be when you are in this Wuji posture.

Chapter 2: The Foundation of Xingyiquan

The Wuji Song of Xingyiquan 形意拳無極歌

One misty Qi, cultivate (it) internally and externally. Jing and Wei rivers not dividing is the natural source of the Dao. Empty and natural, condense your Shen (i.e., spirit) and remain calm. Converting into nothingness and returning to the "origin" come from this.

混淪一氣內外修，涇渭不分至道由。
空洞自然凝神靜，化虛還原此中求。

In Wuji, since Yin and Yang are not distinguished, there is only one Qi. Since this Qi does not have Yin and Yang, it is transparent to the entire universe. When you are in the Wuji state, this Qi can be cultivated so that it fills your body internally and combines with the external, natural Qi around you. It will feel like your body is transparent.

Jing (涇) and Wei (渭) are two rivers. Jing originates in Gansu Province (甘肅省) and its water is muddy. When the Jing enters Shanxi Province (陝西省), it joins the Wei river and the water becomes clear. This means that when you are entering the Wuji state, it should be like the Jing water entering the Wei River and becoming calm and clear, so that no distinction can be made between them. This says that in the Wuji state, there is no distinction between clear and muddy. Everything is empty and natural. In this state, you simply keep your Shen on the spirit center (Upper Dan Tian, 上丹田) and remain calm. When you are able to reach this level, your spirit and feeling will be able to reach the level of nothingness (i.e., absolute clarity). This is the way of the Dao in returning our feelings to their very origin.

The One Qi of Xingyiquan 形意拳一氣

Taiji was originally misty and turbid, no shape, no Yi. But there is one Qi within. This Qi circulates in the universe, nowhere cannot be reached. Living things then originated. Named "One Qi," also called "Pre-Heaven Real Sole Qi."

太極本混混沌沌，無形無意，而其中卻含有一氣，其氣
流行宇內，無所不至，而生機萌焉。名曰〝一氣〞。亦
曰〝先天真一之氣〞。

Taiji (太極) means "grand ultimate" which implies some existing "grand ultimate" power or force in nature or Dao. From this Taiji, Yin and Yang, two poles, are derived from the state of Wuji (無極)(i.e., no extremity) and also makes the Yin-Yang state return to its Wuji state.

When Yin and Yang are discriminated from Wuji state, Yin stands for all that is soft, dark, feminine, passive, internal, etc. Yang stands for all that is hard, bright, masculine, active, external, etc. Everything is partly Yin and partly Yang. Together they form the two poles or extremes between which all of creation lies. As a unit, they are referred to as Taiji, the supreme ultimate or extreme power of the nature.

23

However, before Yin and Yang (two polarities or extremes), there was Wuji (no polarities or extremes). Because there were no extremes or poles by which the character of anything could be distinguished, it is said that the universe was "misty" or "turbid." Naturally, in the state of Wuji there is no shape (no physical form) and no Yi (no intention). However, regardless of whether one is in a state of Wuji or Yin-Yang (tow poles), there is still only one Qi. This Qi may vary, but it is still the same Qi which fills the universe and is responsible for all living things. This Qi is sometimes called the "One Qi" (一氣). It is also called Pre-Heaven Real Qi (先天真一之氣) because it existed even before heaven and earth were distinguished.

> From this Qi, the two poles (Yin and Yang) were generated and the heaven and the earth began to divide. Since then, the Yin and Yang were distinguished. Men were also generated. Therefore, the Qi, as a matter of fact, is the root of man's nature and life, the source of creation and variation, the origin (i.e., determiner) of life and death. (If) men are able to Yang Qi (i.e., nourish Qi) and protect it without loss, then long life. If (men) abuse it and lose it and let it disperse and dissipate, then they die young.

由是氣而生兩儀，而天地始分，陰陽始判，人類亦于是乎產生。故是氣也，實為人類性命之根，造化之源，生死之本。人能養是氣而保之弗失，則長生。漸喪之而聽其渙散，則夭死。

Because of the Qi, Yin and Yang were distinguished. When Yin and Yang interact, millions of lives are created, including men. Yang Qi (養氣) means to keep, protect, nourish, and cultivate the Qi and make it firm and strong. Yang Qi is the main training of Chinese Qigong and the internal martial arts. Since Qi is the root of life and the origin of creation and variation, if you learn how to protect and cultivate it, you are certain to have a long life.

> (To practice) Xingyiquan is to use the Post-Heaven man to train, to comprehend and interact with Yin and Yang, to combine creation and variation; (it is) the desire to turn around heaven and earth, return from Post-Heaven to Pre-Heaven, protect and nourish the Qi, and make possible the ascent to the domain of longevity. Therefore, although the Quan (i.e., Xingyiquan) has millions of variations, hundreds of marvelous tricks, if (we) examine all of them, there is nothing but only "Lian Qi" (i.e., train Qi), two words.

"形意拳"者，是以後天人為之鍛練，參陰陽，合造化，欲旋乾轉坤，由後天返先天，保養是氣，而使之登于壽域者也。故是拳雖變化萬端，玄妙百出，若概括言之，總不外乎"練氣"二字而矣。

Before your birth is called Pre-Heaven (Xian Tian, 先天), because you had not yet seen the sky or heaven. Post-Heaven (Hou Tian, 後天) means after your birth. In order to reverse your progress down the path of aging and physically degenerating (turning around heaven and earth) and return to your origin (Pre-Heaven, childhood), you must understand Yin and Yang and learn how to apply them to your body harmoniously. This will enable you to thoroughly comprehend creation and variation.

Lian Qi (練氣) means to train, to strengthen, and to refine the Qi. Although there are many techniques and variations in Xingyiquan, it is ultimately only a question of training and refining your Qi.

Two Poles of Xingyiquan 形意拳兩儀

Two Poles, originated from one Qi, are heaven and earth. That is Yin and Yang. (If) only Yang, then will not live; (if) only Yin, will not grow. (When) Yin and Yang mutually brew, then millions of lives are born. This is the natural rule of heaven and earth. The human body is also a small heaven and earth. From four limbs and hundreds of bones, every action and every move, not one cannot be distinguished with Yin and Yang. (When) Yin and Yang combine harmoniously, then the body is strong and the movements are smooth. When Yin or Yang is abnormal, then the body is weak and the movements lose their order. This is because Yin and Yang are born from "Pre-Heaven Real Sole Qi." However, in order to raise this Pre-Heaven Real Sole Qi, (to) keep and protect it, (you) must also start from the harmonious regulation of Yin and Yang. Therefore, whoever practices Xingyiquan cannot (gain the essence) without knowing the two poles.

兩儀者，由一氣而生，即天地也，亦即陰陽也。獨陽則
不生，孤陰則不長，陰陽醞釀，而萬物化生，此天地自
然之理也。人生亦一小天地也；凡四肢百骸，一舉一動，
無一不可以陰陽分之。陰陽和，則體健而動作順遂；陰
陽乖，則體弱而舉動失措。蓋陰陽由〝先天真一之氣〞
而生。然欲養此先天真一之氣，而保持不失，亦必先自
陰陽調和始，此習〝形意拳〞者不可不知兩儀者也。

The Chinese consider heaven (Qian, 乾) and earth (Kun, 坤) to be Yang and Yin respectively. When Yin and Yang interact and combine harmoniously, they generate life. All Yin and Yang interactions and variations are generated from one thing, "Pre-Heaven Real Sole Qi" (先天真一之氣). This Qi is also called "Original Qi" (元氣), and it is the Qi you inherit from your parents. Readers who would like to know more about these concepts should refer to *The Root of Chinese Qigong* by Dr. Yang. What is true in the large scale is also true in the small scale, and your body is like a small heaven and earth in that it has Yin and Yang within it. Every part of your body and every movement can also be identified as Yin or Yang. When you know all these aspects of Yin and Yang and understand how to coordinate them harmoniously, you will have grasped the secret of Yin and Yang in Xingyiquan practice.

Using the body as an example, the shoulders are Yang and the hips are Yin. Shoulders and hips must be mutually combined (i.e., coordinated), (then) the Yin and Yang are mutually combined (i.e., harmonized). Elbows are Yang and knees are Yin. Elbows and knees must be mutually combined, (then) Yin and

Yang are mutually combined. Hands are Yang and feet are Yin. Hands and feet must be mutually combined, (then) Yin and Yang are mutually combined. When they are applied in the movements, extension is Yang and withdrawal is Yin. Rise is Yang and fall is Yin. Extending and withdrawing should be natural, rising and falling should be appropriate, then they are the combination (i.e., coordination) of Yin and Yang. In addition, there is Yang within Yin, and Yin within Yang; from the extreme of Yin, Yang is born; and from the extreme of Yang, then Yin is born. (They) interact mutually and generate variations which are hard to figure out. Those learning should comprehend their meaning and clearly distinguish them.

如以人體言：肩，陽也；胯，陰也。肩與胯須相合，即陰陽相合也。肘，陽也；膝，陰也。肘與膝須相合，即陰陽相合也。手，陽也；足，陰也。手與足須相合，即陰陽相合也。以動作言：伸，陽也；縮，陰也；起，陽也，落，陰也。伸縮自然，起落合度，亦即陰陽相合之謂也。他如陰中有陽，陽中有陰，陰極則生陽，陽極則生陰，錯綜變化，莫可端倪，學者須體會其意而明辨之可也。

In Xingyiquan, the shoulders and the hips, the elbows and the knees, the hands and the feet are considered as Yang and Yin respectively. Shoulders and hips combined, elbows and knees combined, and hands and feet combined are called "the three external combinations." Each pair must be coordinated in practice, otherwise you will lose the harmonious coordination of Yin and Yang, and you will also lose the meaning of Xingyiquan.

Yin and Yang also apply to movements. For example, extending is Yang and withdrawing is Yin, etc. Then these moving strategies can be coordinated smoothly and harmoniously, then the Xingyiquan reaches a higher level, and its usefulness for health and defense increase.

Song of Taiji 太極歌

(When) the Xin Monkey (emotional mind) has started to move, the fist and the postures move. Hard and soft, insubstantial and substantial, open, closed, raising and falling.

心猿已動，拳勢斯作，剛柔虛實，開合起落。

In Chinese philosophy, when you are in a state of quiet you are considered to be in a state of "Wuji." Wuji means "no extremities," or "no poles." Since nothing is happening, there is no differentiation between anything. However, once there is an impulse or motion, it is possible to differentiate between parts. You are then in a state called "Taiji," or "supreme ultimate," and everything is divided into Yin and Yang.

In Chinese Qigong society, the monkey is used to represent the mind which is generated from the emotions. The emotional mind is called "Xin" (心), which means "heart." Originally, you are in a state of Wuji, and your mind is empty of thoughts. When you perform or use Xingyiquan in fighting, your emotional mind becomes active and generates an intention. The fist and the postures move according to this intention and emotional feeling. When this happens, the original state of Wuji becomes Yin and Yang. Hard, substantial, open, and rising are Yang; whereas soft, insubstantial, closed, and falling are Yin. Your martial techniques are alive only when you have combined Yin and Yang harmoniously and can exchange them and use their relationship skillfully. From this, we can see that it is the "intention" which makes the Wuji state changed into the state of Yin-Yang, i.e. two poles. This implies that "Taiji" in this action is actually the "mind."

In Xingyiquan, the "three body posture" (see Chapter 4) is considered the derivation of the Taiji concept in the posture. Once you start to move from the standing Wuji state into the three body posture, Yin and Yang are differentiated, and defensive and offensive intentions have been generated.

Xingyi Taiji Song 形意太極歌

Wuji is the mother which bears Yin and Yang. Motion (yields) division, (when) calm, (all is) combined, two poles assist. Within this, Three Powers and Four Phases are all not lost. This is (also) the master of the Five Phases, Six Combinations, and Seven Stars.

無極乃生陰陽母，動分靜合兩儀輔。
三才四象皆無遺，五行六合七曜主。

When Yin and Yang are divided, the two poles become clear. The various techniques and strategies are generated from the coordination of Yin and Yang. The "Three Powers" (San Cai, 三才) originally meant Heaven (Tian, 天), Earth (Di, 地), and Man (Ren, 人). In Xingyiquan however, they refer to the three parts of the body in the three body posture: the head, hands, and feet. This posture is the most basic one in Xingyiquan, and all other movements or strategies originate from it. "Four Phases" (Si Xiang, 四象) originally meant the Four Phases generated from the two poles. In Xingyiquan, the Four Phases refer to body movement, hand techniques, leg techniques, and the stepping strategy. The "Five Phases" (Wu Xing, 五行) in philosophy are metal (Jin, 金), water (Shui, 水), wood (Mu, 木), fire (Huo, 火), and earth (Tu, 土). In Xingyiquan they refer to the five basic techniques: Pi (劈), Zuan (鑽), Beng (弸), Pao (炮), and Heng (横). The "Six Combinations" (Liu He, 六合) in Xingyiquan include mind and body combinations. The mind's combinations are the Xin with the Yi (the emotional mind with the wisdom mind), the Yi with the Qi, and the Qi with the Li (力)(i.e., muscular power). The combinations of the body are the hands with the feet, the elbows with the knees, and the shoulders with the hips. The "Seven Stars" in Xingyiquan are the seven parts of the body: the head, shoulders, elbows, hands, hips, knees, and feet.

Song of Two Poles 兩儀歌

The eagle and bear are competing in the strength of their wills (i.e., fighting), adopt (their) techniques as a Quan (style). Within it, Yin and Yang are combined secretly. (This is) the source of Xingyi.

鷹熊兢志，取法為拳，陰陽暗合，形意之源。

In Xingyiquan, the eagle is considered Yang because it specializes in attacking and advancing, while the bear is considered Yin because it is calm and steady, which is characteristic of defense. In fact, when you stand still and calm before Xingyiquan movement, it is Wuji, and when you move and form the "three body posture" (see Chapter 4), it is the manifestation of Yin and Yang. Later, when the Xingyiquan strategies are performed in continuous movements, the two poles of Yin and Yang start to mutually exchange, interact, and coordinate with each other harmoniously.

Thesis of the Two Poles 兩儀說

The two poles are the postures of eagle and bear in the sequence, are the theory of defense, protection, attacking, control, advancing, and retreating. We men own four limbs and hundreds of bones, (when they are) extended they are Yang (the eagle posture); (when they are) withdrawn they are Yin (the bear posture). Therefore, it is said "Yin and Yang are combined secretly." An ancient wise man who lived deep in the mountains and the distant valley saw an eagle and a bear competing in the strength of their wills (i.e., fighting), and adapted their techniques and created (the Xingyiquan) sequences. Defend and protect like a bear, and attack and advance like an eagle. (If) the forms stray from these two postures, the sequence will lose its reality. It is named "Xingyi" (shape and mind) because it is like their shapes, and the mind imitates their thinking (and feeling).

兩儀者，拳中鷹熊之勢，防守進取往來之理也。吾人俱
有四體百骸，伸之而為陽，縮之而為陰，故曰陰陽暗合
也。先哲在深山窮谷之中，見有鷹熊兢志，因取法為拳。
防守像熊，進取像鷹。越此二勢，其拳失真。名為形意
者，像其形而思其意也。

In this thesis you can see that the most basic movements of Xingyiquan imitate the postures of the eagle when you are attacking and advancing, and the bear when you are protecting your body from attack. The foundation of Xingyiquan was built from imitating the movements (shapes) and the spiritual intentions (Yi) of these two animals. The other ten animal forms are combined and coordinated with these two basic postures and spiritual feelings.

The Three Bodies of Xingyiquan 形意拳三體

The three bodies (are) the phases of the three powers—Heaven, Earth, and Man. In (Xingyiquan) style, they are head, hands, and feet. The three bodies are again divided into three sections and coordinated with each other both internally and externally. The head is the root section. External is the head and internal is the Ni Wan Palace (i.e., dust pill palace). The spine back (thoracic vertebrae) is the middle section, external is the spine back and internal is the heart. The waist is the end section, external is the waist and internal is the (Lower) Dan Tian. Again, similarly, the shoulders are the root section, the elbows are the middle section, and the hands are the end section. The hips are the root section, the knees are the middle section, and the feet are the end section. This means that among the three sections, there are another three sections. This rule matches the number 9 in the six classes. This is what is said in the Daoist Elixir Book: *"the Dao was from the one Qi which originated from nothingness. From this one Qi, Yin and Yang were yielded. From the combination of Yin and Yang, three bodies are formed. When three bodies are born, millions of objects bloom."*

三體者，天地人三才之象也。在拳中為頭手足是也。三體又各分為三節，而內外相合。頭為根節；在外為頭，在內為泥丸宮是也。脊背為中節；在外為脊背，在內為心是也。腰為梢節；在外為腰，在內為丹田是也。又如肩為根節，肘為中節，手為梢節。胯為根節，膝為中節，足為梢節。是三節之中，又各有三節也。此理乃合於六書之九數。丹書云：〝道自虛無生一氣，便從一氣產陰陽，陰陽再合成三體，三體重生萬物張。〞此之謂也。

In Xingyiquan, the entire body is divided into three sections. Each section includes both internal elements, which are related to the internal spiritual cultivation, and external elements, which are related to the external appearance and actions of the physical body. Again, the limbs are divided into three sections in the discussion. The three sections include the root section which generates the power, the middle section which directs the power, and the end section which expresses the power. Ni Wan Gong (泥丸宮)(dust pill palace) is a Daoist term and implies brain or the two glands (pituitary and pineal glands) located at the center of the brain.

According to Chinese belief, the number three is considered a perfect natural number which was given by Heaven. When three is multiplied by three, the structure is round and complete. The number nine was commonly used in the "Six Classes" (Liu Shu, 六書), which are the six basic origins of Chinese characters.

Song of the Three Body Postures 三才歌（三體式）

Among the eight postures, three sections must be clear. Hands, body, and feet. (They) are the central root of the eight postures.

八勢之中，三節宜明，手身及足，八梢中根。

According to the source from which this document was drawn, the eight postures are 1. Ding (頂)(press), 2. Kou (扣)(arc/grab), 3. Yuan (圓)(round), 4. Min (敏)(acute), 5. Bao (抱)(embrace), 6. Chui (垂)(drop), 7. Qu (曲)(bend), and 8. Ting (挺)(thrust). These key words will be discussed later in this section. The three sections are the hands (the end section), the body (the center section), and the feet (the rooting section). In another document, and also in Yue, Fei's three section thesis (Appendix A), the three sections are considered to be the head (top section), the body (middle section), and the legs (bottom section). However, you should not be confused by this apparent conflict. As it is pointed out at the end of Yue, Fei's three section thesis, the body should not be divided into sections, but should work as one unit. The division is made only for the convenience of discussion. In this song, it is obvious that these three sections are adapted to discuss the manifestation of Jin (勁) (internal jerking power). It is said: "The root is at the feet, (Jin is) generated from the legs, controlled by the waist and expressed by the fingers" (*Taijiquan Treatise*, by Zhang, San-Feng, 張三豐). These three sections are the foundation of the correct posture for manifesting Jin.

The Four Techniques of Xingyiquan 形意拳四法

Xingyiquan (has) four techniques, the first is the body techniques, the second is the hand techniques, the third is the leg techniques, and the fourth is the stepping techniques (i.e., stepping strategy).

Body techniques: Should not lean forward or backward. Should not incline to the left or tilt to the right. When (moving) forward, (move) straight forward, and when (retreating) backward, retreat straight backward.

"形意拳"四法，一曰身法，二曰手法，三曰腳法，四曰步法。
身法：不可前栽後仰，不可左斜右歪，往前一直而進，向後一直而退。

Body technique means the strategic movements of the body which set up for manifesting Jin, neutralizing, or occupying the most advantageous position. When you are doing these, the body is upright and does not lean or tilt in any direction. This rule is common to most of the Chinese martial arts styles. In Taijiquan, it is said: "the head is suspended and the tailbone is straight up" (Xu Ling Ding Jin, Weilu Zhong Zeng)(虛領頂勁，尾閭中正). When the body is upright, the spirit can be raised, the legs have a firm root, and the body is able to keep at the center and be balanced.

Xingyiquan is more aggressive than other internal styles, and its main strategy is "using offense as defense" (Yi Gong Wei Shou)(以攻為守). Therefore, from the strategic point of view, straight forward movement is the most important. However, when you are in a disadvantageous situation and you must retreat, you must move quickly straight backward.

> *Hand techniques: Its Jin is in the wrist, its Li is in the fingers. When turning, agile and alive, opening and closing are natural and smooth.*

手法：其勁在腕，其力在指，轉動靈活，開合自如。

Xingyiquan is classified as a soft-hard style. This means that the beginning of a movement is soft, so that the Qi can be led to the extremities easily. This Qi will then be able to energize the muscles and manifest the Jin. Readers interested in studying more about Jin (勁)(martial power) should refer to the book: *Tai Chi Theory and Martial Power*, by Dr. Yang. When you use hands for attacking or defending, the Jin is manifested in the wrist. The wrist must be soft, because that is where the Qi is directed to the fingers. When this Qi is directed to the fingers, the fingers' Li (力)(muscular strength) can be manifested efficiently. The wrist should be able to turn agilely and lively, and the fingers should be able to open and close easily and smoothly.

> *Leg techniques: (When) the leg is raised, it is for Zuan (drill). (When) the leg is landing, the leg is turning. (If) not drilling and not turning, one inch (stepping) ahead.*

腳法：腳起而躜，腳落而翻，不躜不翻，一寸而先。

In Xingyiquan, the straight forward drilling kick is one of the most common. Xingyiquan normally emphasizes short-range fighting, so the kicking is also short-range, and the targets are usually the groin and below, such as the knees and shins. It is hard to make these short kicks powerful, so Xingyiquan uses a drilling motion to increase the penetration and forward strength. That is why it is said: "(When) the leg is raised, it is for Zuan (鑽)(drill)."

If the opponent is able to escape skillfully from your kicks, your drilling kick will have lost its purpose. You should then take advantage of his retreat by turning your leg and stepping forward to again put your opponent in an urgent situation.

If your leg is not used for either kicking or turn stepping forward, you should always keep your stepping strategy one inch ahead of your opponent's. This means that you only need to be one inch ahead of your opponent to have him in a disadvantageous position.

> *Stepping Techniques: There is inch stepping, urgent (or speedy) stepping, drill stepping, three techniques. "Inch stepping" is extending the body and using the inch power to urge and force (the body) to advance. The rear leg is bounced, the front foot automatically (steps) forward. "Urgent stepping' is the horse-shaped step. Its key is all in the rear leg's power. It is said, all of the message (power) relies on the bounce of the rear leg. In "drill stepping," the front leg steps straight forward and the rear foot follows. (Of) the stepping techniques, overshadowing the "inch" and the "urgent" stepping, the "drill stepping' is the most common and is the most important among the three.*

步法：又有寸步，疾步，躦步三法。寸步者，即張身用
寸力催逼而進，後足一蹬，前足自進。疾步者，馬形步
也。其要全在後足用力，所謂消息全憑後足蹬也。躦步
者，一足放直前進，後足隨之。步法除寸疾二步外，躦
步最為普通，在三步中尤稱最要者也。

The last important area in Xingyiquan is the stepping. Proper positioning and speed can put you in the most advantageous position to execute your techniques. There are three common stepping strategies. The first one is the "inch stepping" (Cun Bu, 寸步) which was mentioned earlier. In inch stepping, the rear leg is used to push the front leg forward an inch at a time. This is commonly used when you are already in an advantageous situation and you would like to keep your opponent in a sealed and urgent position. You use inch stepping when you are close and do not have enough time to change your feet (i.e., to step the other foot forward).

"Urgent stepping" (Ji Bu, 疾步) is like the movement of a horse. The rear leg thrusts backward to propel the front leg forward. This is commonly used to chase the opponent and to shorten the range. It is usually used in coordination with hand techniques. In urgent stepping you usually push with the back leg and step forward with the front leg, though if you need to cover more ground you can then also step forward with the rear leg.

"Drill stepping" (Zuan Bu, 躦步) is not "drill kicking." To use drill stepping, you have to keep looking for a gap in the opponent's posture or an "empty door" (Kong Men, 空門). "Empty door" is a martial arts term which refers to an area where the opponent is open to attack. When you see an opening you step in with your front leg, and then follow with your rear leg. In other words, if your right leg is forward, you step forward with your right leg, and then bring up your left leg the same distance so that your legs are not too far apart. An alternative stepping is to step forward with your rear (left) leg and then "follow" with your right leg (i.e., bring it up so that your legs are not too far apart). With this stepping you use your front leg like a drill and drill into any weaknesses you find in your enemy's position. The movement is just like a butterfly flying among the flowers, agile and alive. Drill stepping is the most common and most important stepping in Xingyiquan.

Song of Four Phases 四象歌

Already completing four fists training, (techniques must) vary following the opportunity. Calm like a mountain, move like the collapse of a mountain.

已成四拳，隨機應變，靜如山岳，動如崩翻。

"Quan" (拳) literally means "fist," but is also can mean "style" or "technique." Here it means "basic techniques." The text following this song in the original document explains that the four basic techniques are: the head punch (Tou Quan, 頭拳) (i.e., hand strikes). It is called this because the hand is the "head" of the punch.), pluck and lead (Tiao Ling, 挑領), eagle's seizing (Ying Zhuo, 鷹捉), and sticky hands (Zhan Shou, 沾手).

After you have mastered these four basic Xingyiquan techniques, then they must be alive and agile in corresponding with the opponent's movements. You need also to catch the right opportunity and use the right timing in applying them. Only when you are confident in these can your mind be calm and centered. When you are still, you are steady and calm like a mountain both internally and externally. Once you start to move, the power from your calm and concentrated mind can be as great as the collapse of a mountain.

The Jin of the Four Extremities 四梢勁

The four extremities are the tongue, teeth, nails, and hair. The tongue is the extremity of the meat (muscles), the teeth are the extremities of the bones, the nails are the extremities of the tendons, and the hair is the extremity of the blood. The four extremities must be uniform. The method of uniformity is as if the tongue is crushing the teeth, as if the teeth are breaking the tendons, as if the nails are penetrating the bones, and as if the hair is pushing up the hat. The heart (decides) for a war, then internally starts to act. The Qi is generated from the Dan Tian. Like the fury of the tiger, like the alertness of the dragon, Qi is emitted following the sound, the sound is emitted following the hands (techniques). When the sound is falling, the hand is falling (i.e., the technique is completed). One branch moves, hundreds of branches shake. The four extremities are unified, then no internal Jin will not be emitted.

四梢者，舌牙甲髮是也。舌為肉梢，牙為骨梢，甲為筋梢，髮為血梢，四梢要齊。至於齊之之法，舌若摧齒，牙若斷筋，甲若透骨，髮若沖冠。心一戰，而內舉動。氣自丹田生，如虎之恨，如龍之驚，氣發隨聲，聲隨手發，手隨聲落。一枝動，百枝搖，四梢無不齊，內勁無不出也。

Qi is the main source of Jin, and Jin occurs when Qi is manifested in the extremities. Therefore, "Jin" here means the "manifestation of Qi." When Qi can be manifested in these four extremities, then the Qi will be full and be able to reach every tiny place in the body. This article is followed by a thesis which discusses the Jin of these four extremities.

Thesis of the Four Extremities 四梢說

The extremities of a man's blood, meat (muscles), tendons, and bones are called "Shao" (endings). That is, the hair is the extremity of the blood, the tongue is the extremity of the meat (muscle), the teeth are the extremities of the bones, and the claws (i.e., nails) are the extremity of the tendons. When the these four extremities manifest their strength, they are able to change their normal state and frighten people.

人之血肉筋骨之末端曰梢。蓋髮為血梢，舌為肉梢，牙
為骨梢，爪為筋梢。四梢用力，則可變其常態，能使人
生畏懼焉。

The end of anything is called "Shao" (梢). In Chinese medicine and Qigong, it is believed that your state of health is reflected in the condition of your extremities. A doctor can judge your health and form a diagnosis by examining your hands and feet. A Qigong master can tell if your Qi is abundant by checking whether it has reached the extremities. Thousands of years of experience have shown that the hair is closely related to the blood, and can show the condition of the blood. In the same way, the tongue, teeth, and nails are related respectively to the muscle, bones, and tendons.

Because of all these relationships, Xingyiquan emphasizes training which leads Qi to these four extremities. If the Qi is able to reach these endings, then the Qi in the body will naturally be abundant and the power generated from this internal energy will be very great. When this power is manifested in these four extremities, it can change their normal appearance (e.g., the hair will stick up) and scare the opponent.

The first is the blood extremity: The angry Qi fills up the chest, the hair sticks up and raises the hat. The circulation of the blood speeds up. The opponent will automatically feel scared. Though the hairs are tiny, it is not difficult to destroy the opponent.

一・血梢：怒氣填胸，豎髮衝冠，血輪速轉，敵膽自寒，
髮毛雖微，摧敵不難。

In order to make the Qi reach the hair, which is the extremity of the blood, you must first have plenty of oxygen to energize the blood to a higher state. Blood cells are the carriers of Qi and oxygen. When blood cells are raised to a higher energy level, the Qi will reach the hair. You have probably heard people say that someone was so mad that his hair was sticking up. This can actually happen if his emotion raises the energy level of the blood enough so that the Qi is able to reach to the ends of the hair. Scientists believe that Qi might be what is called "bioelectricity." This would explain the phenomenon, because when the hairs are electrically charged they will repel each other and stick up. For more information on the modern explanation of Qi, please refer to Dr. Yang's book, *The Root of Chinese Qigong*.

The second is the meat (muscle) extremity: The tongue is curled and the Qi is sunk. Even the mountain will be shaking. (When) the meat is raised up, it is like iron. The spirit of vitality is raised and the bravery is built. (Just) one word, and its sternness can make the opponent's vigor fail, and he loses his bravery.

二‧肉梢：舌捲氣降，雖山亦撼，肉豎似鐵，精神勇敢，
一言之威，落魄喪膽。

"Meat" (Rou, 肉) refers to the muscles. It is believed that the tongue is closely related to the muscles. If the tongue is curved upward to touch the roof of the mouth, it will close the circuit between the Conception and Governing Vessels (Ren and Du Mai, 任、督脈) and allow the free circulation of Qi through them. This also allows Qi to be built up. If you let this Qi sink to and accumulate in the Lower Dan Tian below your navel, it will energize the muscles to a very high level. This Qi will be so strong that it will seem to be able to shake a mountain. When this Qi fills your muscles, they will feel inflated or "raised," and they will be as strong as iron. The higher energy level will also raise your spirit of vitality and make you braver. Then, just one word from you will strike fear into the heart of your enemy.

The third is the bone extremity: There is a bravery in the bones. When biting the teeth, then (Jin can be) emitted. The opponent's meat can be eaten, the fury is able to make the eyes pop out. All of these are the achievement of the teeth, which will drive the opponent to distraction.

三‧骨梢：有勇在骨，切齒則發，敵肉可食，眥裂目突，
惟齒之功，令人恍惚。

When people are furious, they sometimes bite their teeth together very hard. This comes from our animal ancestry. When we are fighting mad, the emotion enables the Qi to reach the bones. This Qi goes to the teeth, and prepares them for biting our enemy. When you are mad enough to virtually eat your opponent, your eyes also bulge out. If you are able to do all this in front of an opponent, you will scare him so much that he will lose all thought of fighting.

The fourth is the tendon extremity: The tiger (is) awe-inspiring and the eagle fierce, use the claw as the sharp point, the hands seize and the legs step, the Qi is vehement and abundant; where the claw reaches, all things can be accomplished.

四‧筋梢：虎威鷹猛，以爪為鋒，手攫足踏，氣勢兼雄，
爪之所到，皆可湊功。

This last part of the song says that when the Qi is strong and abundant, the nails, which are related to the tendons, can be as powerful as the claws of the tiger or eagle. This song also emphasize the awe-inspiring feeling of a tiger and the calm but sharp spirit of the eagle. When you have these two spirits and the strong Qi which can reach the nails, then there is nothing that you cannot accomplish.

Five Basic Patterns of Xingyiquan 形意拳五綱

Pi Quan belongs to Metal in the Five Phases; it is able to nourish the lungs. If its Jin is smooth, the lung Qi will be harmonious. Because man is mastered by Qi, when Qi is harmonious, then the body is naturally strong.

劈拳者，五行屬金而養肺。其勁順，則肺氣和。夫人以
氣為主，氣和則體自壯也。

Pi (劈), Zuan (鑽), Beng (弸), Pao (炮), and Heng (橫) are the five most basic patterns of Xingyiquan. It is very difficult to find English words which exactly correspond to them and express both the feeling and the movement accurately. Pi can mean split, rend, or cleave. However, some of these words have lost the feeling of the actual action (attacking), while others have lost the feeling of tearing apart. When doing Pi, the front hand is formed like an ax and chops down on something. However, in the actual movement, the chopping force is not exactly downward; instead, it is forward and downward. But you are also making a motion as if you were using both hands to rend or tear apart something. For example, when applying Pi you may use your left hand to grab the opponent's wrist, and place your right hand on his shoulder area and chop downward. This will tear the shoulder apart and dislocate it. Pi (and each of the other four patterns) is a pattern of movement to express Jin, instead of a specific action. Pi can be any one of several movements, but it must always have its characteristic pattern or feeling through which the Jin is manifested.

In Xingyiquan, the five basic patterns are related to the Five Phases of Chinese philosophy and medicine, and have the same interrelationships. These Five Phases are Metal (Jin, 金), Water (Shui, 水), Wood (Mu, 木), Fire (Huo, 火), and Earth (Tu, 土). Therefore, these five basic patterns are also commonly called the "Wu Xing" (五行)(Five Phases) or "Wu Quan" (五拳)(Five Fists). It is believed that the movements of each of these five patterns benefits the health of the related internal organ. We will discuss this in more detail in Chapter 4. Pi is considered to belong to Metal, and is able to nourish the lungs. If the Qi is smooth when you emit Pi Jin, then the lung Qi will be harmonious.

Zuan Quan belongs to Water in the Five Phases; it is able to nourish the kidneys. The flowing of its Qi is like the water flowing in the curve (i.e., river), nowhere will not be reached. When its Qi is harmonious, then the kidneys are firm, the clean Qi will rise and the dirty Qi will sink.

鑽拳者，五行屬水，能補腎。其氣之行，如水之曲曲而
流，無微不至也。其氣和，則腎足，清氣上升，濁氣下
降。

The Chinese word "Zuan" (鑽) has the meaning of drilling, penetrating, and forcing one's way through. The motion is straight forward, aggressive, and rotating like a drill. Though the motion is forward, it is usually also upward or downward. In Xingyiquan, the Zuan moving pattern belongs to Water in the Five Phases. The Qi circulates like water flowing in a curved river: smooth, and reaching every tiny area. When the Qi circulation is smooth and harmonious, the Qi in the kidneys can be regulated. In addition, practicing Zuan can raise the clean Qi and sink the dirty Qi.

Beng Quan belongs to Wood in the Five Phases; it is able to ease the liver, and is the stretching and withdrawing of the one Qi. When its fist is smooth, then the liver will be peaceful and the spirit of vitality will grow; (it is also) able to strengthen the tendons and bones (i.e., physical body), and enhance the condition of the brain.

崩拳者，五行屬木，能舒肝，是一氣之伸縮也。其拳順，
則肝平而長精神，強筋骨，壯腦力。

The Chinese word "Beng" (崩) means stretching, developing, extending, and powerfully expanding. It feels like a strong bow which has been stretched, and whose power is able to crush anything. In Xingyiquan, the Beng moving pattern belongs to Wood in the Five Phases. It is like a tree which can grow and be bent like a bow. The Qi in this pattern extends and withdraws. When the Beng movement is smooth, it can benefit the Qi circulation of the liver. Furthermore, this movement can raise the spirit of vitality, strengthen the physical body, and supply plenty of Qi nourishment to the brain.

Pao Quan belongs to Fire in the Five Phases; it is an opening and closing of the one Qi. (It is) like the explosion of a cannon. When its Qi is harmonious, then within the heart will be light and agile, the body will be comfortable and invigorated.

炮拳者，五行屬火，能養心，是一氣之開合，如炮炸裂
也。其氣和，則心中虛靈，身體舒暢。

The Chinese word "Pao" (炮) has the sense of an explosion, like a cannon shooting a cannon ball. The power is straight forward, strong, fast, and destructive. In the Five Phases, the Pao moving pattern belongs to Fire, and is related to the heart. In the Pao movement, the Qi either is closed and remains quiet, or opens like an explosion, fast and powerful. When the Pao movement is smooth, the stagnant Qi stored in the body can be released and emitted from the body. For example, when you are depressed and your Qi is stagnant, if you suddenly stand up, shout, and punch a few times, you will feel much better and more comfortable. This movement will help release the Fire accumulated in the heart. Your body will feel comfortable and natural, and you will be able to move around easily.

Heng Quan belongs to Earth; it is able to nourish the spleen and harmonize the stomach. (It is) the gathering of the one Qi. Its shape is round and its characteristic is solid. When its Qi is smooth, then the Five Phases will be harmonious and hundreds of lives will be produced.

橫拳者，五行屬土，能養脾和胃，是一氣之團聚也。其
形圓，其性實，其氣順，則五行和而百物生焉。

The word "Heng" (橫) means to cross, move sideways, or to force through aggressively with a sideward motion. It also has the sense of two forces moving in opposite directions to balance each other. In the Five Phases, this movement belongs to Earth, and is related to the spleen and the stomach. This movement is able to make the Qi gathered at its center (i.e., between the solar plexus and the navel) round and full. When the Qi is smooth from doing the Heng movement, then the other four Qis will coordinate with each other harmoniously.

> *The shape of Pi Quan is like an ax, therefore it belongs to Metal. The appearance of Zuan Quan is like thunder, therefore it belongs to Water. The aspect of Beng Quan is like an arrow, therefore it belongs to Wood. The appearance of Pao Quan is like a cannon, therefore it belongs to Fire. The configuration of Heng Quan is like a ball, it therefore belongs to Earth. From the theory of mutual production, Pi Quan is able to generate Zuan Quan, Zuan Quan is able to produce Beng Quan, Beng Quan is able to yield Pao Quan, Pao Quan is able to generate Heng Quan, and finally Heng Quan is able to produce Pi Quan. From the theory of mutual conquest, Pi Quan is able to conquer Beng Quan, Beng Quan is able to defeat Heng Quan, Heng Quan is able to suppress Zuan Quan, Zuan Quan is able to conquer Pao Quan, and Pao Quan is able to defeat Pi Quan.*

> 劈拳之形似斧，故屬金。鑽拳之形似電，故屬水。弸拳之形似箭，故屬木。炮拳之形似炮，故屬火。橫拳之形似彈，故屬土。由相生之理論之，劈拳能生鑽拳，鑽拳能生弸拳，弸拳能生炮拳，炮拳能生橫拳，橫拳能生劈拳。由相克之理論之，劈拳能克弸拳，弸拳能克橫拳，橫拳能克鑽拳，鑽拳能克炮拳，炮拳能克劈拳。

This section explains why the five basic moving patterns correspond to the Five Phases. Like the Five Phases, they also follow the pattern of mutual production and conquest. We will discuss these relationships in more detail in Chapter 5.

The Song of Five Jins 五勁歌

> *After understanding the three sections, the five Jins mutually assist (each other). Cai (stepping), Pu (leap), Guo (enwrapping), and Shu (binding)(i.e., sealing), especially Jue (thrusting), which should not be misunderstood.*

> 三節明後，五勁相佐，踩撲裹束，惟決勿錯。

Once you comprehend the real meaning of the three sections, you should then try to understand the five basic Jins of Xingyiquan.

> *The Five Jins, Cai (stepping), Pu (leap), Guo (enwrapping), Shu (binding)(i.e., sealing), and Jue (thrusting). Cai Jin (Stepping Jin) is like stepping on something poisonous. Pu Jin (Leaping Jin) is like the leaping of the rabbit and the tiger. Guo Jin (Enwrapping Jin) is like wrapping something so that nothing is exposed. Shu Jin (Binding Jin) is like binding the top and the bottom into one. Jue Jin (Thrusting Jin) is like water breaking through a dam. The Stepping needs the*

Thrusting, the Leaping needs the Thrusting, the Enwrapping needs the Thrusting, The Thrusting needs the Thrusting. One Thrusting, not one without thrust. If there is no thrusting, there is no agility.

五勁者，踩撲裏束決。踩勁如踩毒物也。撲勁如兔虎之
撲也。裏勁如裏物而不露也。束勁如上下束而為一也。
決勁如水決也。踩要決，撲要決，裏要決，束要決，決
要決。一決而無不決，非決而不靈也。

This paragraph explains the five Jins (Cai, Pu, Guo, Shu, Jue; 踩、撲、裏、束、決) with examples which give you the actual feeling of these Jins and the movements through which they manifest. Among these five, the most important is the thrusting Jin. Thrusting means fast and powerful actions. It is so basic and essential that the other four Jins must also manifest it so that they will be agile and powerful.

About Five Phases 五行說

The Five Phases are Metal, Wood, Water, Fire, and Earth. (It is) like a man who has five viscera internally and five organs externally. All (of these) are matched with the Five Phases. The heart belongs to Fire, the spleen belongs to Earth, the liver belongs to Wood, the lungs belong to Metal, and the kidneys belong to Water. These are the Five Phases which are hidden internally. The eyes are connected to the liver, the nose is connected with the lungs, the tongue is connected to the heart, the ears are connected with the kidneys, and the Renzhong is connected with the spleen. These are the Five Phases which appear on the outside. There is a Dao of mutual production among the Five Phases. Metal generates Water, Water generates Wood, Wood generates Fire, Fire generates Earth (ashes), and Earth generates Metal. (They) also have the meaning (i.e., relationships) of mutual conquest. Metal conquers Wood, Wood conquers Earth, Earth conquers Water, Water conquers Fire, and Fire conquers Metal. The Five Phases were seen in the book of Hong Fan, *and were explained in the Confucian books in the Han. Later people have scoffed at their meaning and (said) nothing can be adopted. Therefore, the Dao of mutual production and conquest have been misused. The (Xingyi) Quan adopts them as its name and uses them to strengthen and solidify the internal and modify (i.e., improve) the external. It adopts the theory of mutual production and uses it in the regular practice to strengthen the body and enhance the growth of the Qi and Li. (This is) to prepare for its use in battle. It adopts the meaning (i.e., theory) of mutual conquest to be used for resisting the opponent.*

五行者，金木水火土之謂也。如人之內有五臟，外有五
官，皆與五行相配合。心屬火，脾屬土，肝屬木，肺屬
金，腎屬水，此五行之隱於內者。目通肝，鼻通肺，舌
通心，耳通腎，人中通脾，此五行之著於外者。五行有
相生之道存焉。金生水，水生木，木生火，火生土，土
生金。又有相克之意在焉。金克木，木克土，土克水，
水克火，火克金。夫五行見於洪範，而漢儒藉之解經。
後人每譏其於義無取而生克之道，究不為不當也。拳因
之以名，用以堅實其內，整飾其外，取相生之道，以為
平時之練習，強健其身體，增長其氣力，以備戰時之應
用，取相克之義，以為對敵之抵抗。

This document explains that there are five internal and five external organs which correspond to the Five Phases: Metal, Wood, Water, Fire, and Earth, and these five organs also follow the theory of mutual production and conquest. Renzhong (Gv-26)(人中) is the name of a cavity which is located under the nose and above the upper lip (Figure 2-1). "Hong Fan" (洪範)("The Great Plan") is the title of one section of the *Book of History* (*Shi Ji*, 史記). The relationships of the Five Phases were also explained during the Han Dynasty (漢朝)(206 B.C.-220 A.D.). However, because few people could understand their real meaning, these relationships are frequently misused.

The Six Unifications of Xingyiquan 形意拳六合

(In) Xingyiquan, the most important point is one word—unification. When the movements are unified, then the postures are accurate and gain the advantage. (When) the movements are not unified, then the postures are strange (i.e., abnormal) and the Qi and Li will be in vain. (You) must know this. What is called the "unification" includes six. The body is not leaning, the Xin (emotional mind)

Renzhong (Gv-26)

Figure 2-1. Renzhong cavity

is peaceful and the Qi is harmonious, the Yi (wisdom mind) is not on other matters (i.e., is concentrated), the movements are natural. Then it is called the Xin and the Yi unified, the Yi and the Qi unified, and the Qi and Li unified. These are the three internal unifications.

形意拳最重要之點，在一合字。動作合，則姿勢正而獲
其益。動作不合，則姿勢乖而氣力徒勞。不可不知也。
所謂合者有六。身無偏倚，心平氣和，意不他動，動作
自然，謂之心與意合，意與氣合，氣與力合。此內三合
也。

The "six unifications" (Liu He, 六合) are frequently translated as the "six combinations." The process doesn't just happen by itself. In the beginning, your mind has to make it happen. However, after you have practiced them for a long time, you should be able to do them automatically, without consciously paying attention. The six unifications are divided into three internal and three external unifications. The external unifications enable the entire body to move as one unit, so that the rooting, stability, balance, and the manifestation of Jin can be natural and powerful. The three internal unifications coordinate the emotional mind (Xin, 心) and the wisdom mind (意) with each other so that you can judge accurately. Only when you observe all of these unifications will your Yi be able to lead the Qi to the muscles in order to energize them to a more efficient level.

During movement, (when) both hands have grabbing Jin and the heels of the two feet have the external twisting Jin, it is said that the hands and the feet are unified. (When) the two elbows are sinking and the two knees are locked internally, it is called the elbows and the knees are unified. (When) the two shoulders are relaxed and open in drawing the Jin and the two hips are firmed internally to draw the Jin, it is called the shoulders and the hips are unified. These are the three external unifications. The total is called "the six unifications."

動作時，兩手扣勁，兩足後根向外扭勁，是曰手與足合；
兩肘往下垂勁，兩膝往裡扣勁，是曰肘與膝合；兩肩鬆
開抽勁，兩胯裡根抽勁，是曰肩與胯合。此外三合也。
總名之曰六合。

This section explains the three external unifications. However, you should always remember that in all of these unifications, one part is classified as Yin while the other is classified as Yang. Yin is the root and the source of Yang. Yin grows Yang and Yang manifests Yin. When Yin is strong the Yang can be firm and powerful, and when Yin is weak the Yang will also be weak and will not last long. For example, in the three internal unifications, first the Yi (wisdom mind) is Yin while the Xin (emotional mind) is Yang. When the Yi is strong, the Xin can be controlled directly. Then the Yi is Yin and the Qi is Yang. When the Yi is strong, the Qi can be led efficiently. Finally, Qi is Yin when compared with Li. Qi is internal energy while Li is the external manifestation.

Similarly, the hips are Yin while the shoulders are Yang, the knees are Yin while the elbows are Yang, and the feet are Yin and the hands are Yang. The reason for this is very simple: the legs are the root of the manifestation of Jin, and without the support of the Yin, the Jin will be ineffective and weak.

> *(If) the learner is able to become familiar with the techniques of these six unifications, then when practicing, (he) will automatically understand others which belong to the same category. Then, every movement will not but match the (right) way. In addition to the three internal unifications, one still needs the Xin and the eyes to unify, the liver and the tendons to unify, the spleen and the meat (i.e., muscles) to unify, the lungs and the body to unify, and the kidneys and the bones to unify. In addition to the three external unifications, one still needs the head and the hands to unify, the hands and the body to unify, the body and the stepping to unify. From these, it is known that among the movements in Xingyiquan, no matter if it is internal or external, all have the Yin and Yang discrimination. That means they all conform with the theory of mutual connection. Learners should comprehend this completely.*

> 學者能熟知六合之法，則練習時自能觸類旁通，而一舉
> 一動，無不合法。蓋內三合之外，還須心與眼合，肝與
> 筋合，脾與肉合，肺與身合，腎與骨合；外三合之外，
> 尚須頭與手合，手與身合，身與步合也。觀此可知形意
> 拳動作之間，無論內外，莫不有陰陽之分，即莫不寓有
> 互相聯合之理，學者當體會及之。

Only after you understand the principle of unification, and have mastered it in your techniques, will you be able to grasp the real keys and the essence of Xingyiquan. Once you have reached this stage, then many other things which should be unified in the practice will automatically unify. All of these unifications are based on the theory of Yin and Yang. Again, always remember Yin is the root and the foundation of Yang, and Yang is the manifestation of Yin. When Yin is solid and firm, the manifestation of Yang will be strong. They are connected and cannot be separated.

The Song of Six Unifications 六合歌

The body forms the six postures: chicken legs and dragon body, bear shoulders and eagle's claws, embrace like a tiger, and sound like the thunder.

身成六式，雞腿龍身，熊膀鷹爪，虎抱雷聲。

This text is drawn from a different source than the previous selection. You adopt the postures, movement, and spirit of the five animals, as well as the speed and power of thunder.

The Seven Speeds of Xingyiquan 形意拳七疾

The seven speeds are: the eyes are speedy, the hands are speedy, the feet are speedy, the Yi is speedy, the attack is speedy, advancing and withdrawing are speedy, the body's movements are speedy. Those who learn this fist (Xingyiquan), are required (to master) these seven speeds, then (they are) able to win completely. This is what is called up-down, sideways, forward and backward, the (opponent's) eyes are slower than speedy movements. It is like a living dragon and tiger, it cannot be figured out.

七疾者，眼要疾，手要疾，腳要疾，意要疾，出勢要疾，
進退要疾，身法要疾也。習拳者具此七疾，方能完全制
勝。所謂縱橫往來，目不及瞬，有如生龍活虎，令人不
可捉摸者，唯持此耳。

Seven things must move and react quickly in Xingyiquan in order for you to win a fight. If they all have the proper speed, then your reactions and movements will be agile and lively like the dragon and tiger, and your opponent will not be able to perceive them well enough to understand what you are doing.

First, the eyes must be speedy. The eyes are the sprout of the Xin. The eyes inspect the opponent's emotions, which reach to the Xin. Then (you are) able to respond to the opponent and have variations (i.e., adaptability), gaining victory and success. The document says: "the Xin is the marshal and the eyes are the vanguards." What this says is the Xin is the master which must rely on the eyes' slow or speedy response, so it can vary with the target.

一‧眼要疾。眼為心之苗，目察敵情，達之於心，然後
能應敵變化，取勝成功。譜云：＂心為元帥，眼為先
鋒。＂蓋言心之主宰，均持眼之遲疾而轉移也。

Your eyes are the first part of you to make contact with the opponent in a fight. This contact allows your heart (Xin) to respond. Your Xin is the master, while the eyes go on ahead to determine what is happening. Following the clear judgement of your Yi, your strategy can be varied in adapting to the different situations. Therefore, if your eyes can be speedy in their response to the opponent's movement, the Xin will be able to react quickly, and the Yi can judge the situation immediately. In any decision, Xin and Yi must work closely with each other, the two words are often combined into one word: Xin-Yi (心意). Although sometimes only one of the two words is used to refer to the mind, both concepts must in fact be involved.

Second, the hands must be speedy. The hands are a man's wings. Whenever defending, protecting, advancing, and attacking, all rely on (them). However, the Dao of exchanging hands (i.e., fighting) entirely depends on the slow and fast. The slow one is defeated and the speedy one wins. This is a natural reason. Therefore, it is said: "When the eyes are acute and the hands are fast there is winning; and without, losing." It is also said: "When the hands are raised, they are like arrows; and when they fall, it is like the wind. To chase the wind and run after the moon, do not rest." This means the hand techniques are acute and fast, use the opportunity to attack when the opponent is not prepared. Seize the opponent when he is not expecting it. Do not be afraid if the opponent's body is big and his Li is strong. If I can release my hands like the wind, then (I) will be able to win.

二·手要疾。手者，人之羽翼也。凡扞蔽進攻，無不賴
之。但交手之道，全持遲速，遲者負，速者勝，理之自
然。故俗云："眼明手快，有勝無敗。"譜云："手起
如箭落如風，追風趕月不放鬆。"亦謂手法敏疾，趁其
無備而攻之，出其不意而取之，不怕敵之身大力猛，我
能出手如風，即能勝之也。

Hands are the main weapon in a fight. When your hands can move fast, you may defend yourself and attack the opponent effectively. However, you must understand that the speed of the hand's movement and reactions does not rely only upon the extension and contraction of the muscles. First, the eyes must make contact, the Xin must feel (respond to the information), and the Yi must form a judgement, then the order is given to the appropriate muscles to make the hand move.

The third is the feet must be speedy. The feet are the foundation of the body. When the feet stand steady then the body can be steady. When the feet move forward, the body will follow. In Xingyiquan, the entire body's Li should be transported uniformly and no one place is especially emphasized. When the feet move forward the body will also move forward to occupy the opponent's (disadvantageous) position, then the opponent will fall automatically. It is said: "When the feet are striking and treading on, do not hesitate. The message is to rely entirely on the rear leg's kick (i.e., push), the foot steps in the center door and occupies the (advantageous) position, then even a spiritual opponent has difficulty defending." It is also said: 'The feet are striking seven and the hands are striking three." From this, (we can see that) the feet's speed should be more speedy than the hands' speed.

三·腳要疾。腳者，身體之基也。腳立穩則身穩，腳前
進則身隨之。形意拳中渾身運力平均，無一處偏重，腳
進身進，直槍敵人之位，則彼自仆。譜云："腳打踮意
莫容情，消息全憑後足蹬，腳踏中門槍地位，就是神手
也難防。"又曰："腳打七分手打三。"由是觀之，腳
之疾更當疾於手之疾也。

The feet have two main uses in a fight. One is kicking, and the other is for moving your body into a position which is strategically advantageous. When your kicks are fast, they will be effective, and when you can move fast and occupy the most advantageous position, you will put the opponent in an urgent, defensive position, and put yourself in the best position for attacking or withdrawing. You can see that the speed of your legs can make a significant difference in a battle. In addition to this, your legs are the root and foundation of your body. Without this foundation, your Jin will not have a root, and will necessarily be weak.

The fourth is the Yi must be speedy. The Yi is the marshal of the body. Since we have said that the eyes have the refined ability to examine, the hands have the ability to repel and turn, and the feet have the ability to display their power;

however, their delaying, speed, urgency, and slowness all rely on the Yi's decision. That is what is called "when the Yi is firmed instantly, the eyes, hands, and feet must all follow the key (decision)." Therefore, if the eyes are able to detect even the slightest change, this comes from the Yi. When the hands are released (for striking) and do not come back in vain, it is caused by the Yi. That the feet are able to move fast is also because the Yi makes them move fast. From this, then (we) know that the Yi cannot but be speedy.

四‧意要疾。意者，體之帥也。既言眼有監察之情，手
有轉撥之能，腳有行逗之功，然其遲速緊慢，均惟意之
適從。所謂立意一疾，眼與手腳均得其要領。故眼之明
察秋毫，意使之也；手出不空回，意使之也；腳之捷，
亦意使之捷也。觀乎此，則意之不可不疾可知矣。

Although the speed of the entire physical body is important, the Yi is still the all-important marshal which decides which reactions and strategy to take. If your Yi is uncertain, and slow to respond to an attack, then your strategy will not be firm and your reaction will be slow. This means that your hands and feet will also be slow, since their movements are generated from the Yi. However, you should understand that the Yi should not react in a passive manner. It also plays the main role in directing the eyes to increase their potential for inspection and reaction. When your Yi is firm and your spirit is high, every part of your body will be able to respond agilely to the opponent's strategy.

The fifth is the manifestation of the postures must be speedy. The reason is because what is hidden inside is Yi and what is expressed outside are the postures. When the Yi is speedy, the manifested posture must also be speedy. Whenever there is a change, the postures must be generated from the Yi, and the strategy changed in accordance with the (opponent's) change. This will make it possible that the opponent cannot defeat (you), like (when) there is thunder and (he is) not fast enough to cover his ears, (he is) alarmed and disordered, and does not know the strategy for handling the situation. Then, you will be able to defeat the opponent. If the Yi's change can be very speedy, but the posture's speed cannot follow, then the matching with (the opponent) will be stagnant, and (you) will lose for sure. Therefore, when the Yi and the postures are mutually combined, success can be confirmed. When the Yi is fast and the postures are slow, there is no doubt (you will be) defeated. The practitioners must therefore pay more attention to this.

五‧出勢要疾。夫存乎內者為意，現乎外者為勢。意既
疾矣，出勢更不可不疾也。事變當前，必勢隨意生，隨
機應變，令敵人迅雷不及掩耳，張惶失措，無對待之策，
方能制勝。若意變甚速，而勢疾不足以隨之，則應對乖
張，其敗必矣。故意勢相合，成功可決，意疾勢緩，必
負無疑。習技者可不加之意乎。

The speed of the postures refers to three things. The first is the postures which store (i.e., accumulate) Jin, the second is the postural coordination of the entire body, and the third is the postures which emit the Jin. In a fight, after your Yi has decided what to do, regardless of whether the decision is to defend or to attack, your

Jin (either neutralizing or attacking) first has to be stored. The power with which your Jin manifests is determined by the effectiveness with which you store power in your Yi, Qi, and posture. Even if you have a fast Yi and smooth Qi, if you do not utilize a posture which stores Jin like a bow, then your Jin will still not be powerful. How effective this Jin is depends on how fast you can store it. In the final analysis, the effectiveness of your Jin storage comes from the perfect coordination of every part of your body. If this coordination is slow and disordered, then the Jin you emit will not be powerful and effective.

The sixth is advancing and retreating must be speedy. What this section discusses is the techniques of moving sideways, to and fro, advancing, retreating, and dodging sidewards. When (you) should advance, then advance. Try the best and advance forward. When (you) should retreat, then retreat. Lead the Qi to return (to its origin). About the proper time of advancing and retreating, then (you) must inspect the opponent's strengths and weaknesses. When (he) is strong, then avoid (confrontation) and use wisdom to win. When (he) is weak, then attack, and this can be won by Li. The advancing and retreating must be fast and do not allow the opponent to catch any gap (i.e., chance or opening). This is what is called: "High and low following the time (i.e., opportunity), vertical and horizontal following the situation."

六・進退要疾。此節所論，乃縱橫往來進退反側之法也。
當進則進，竭其力而直前。當退則退，領其氣而回轉。
至進退之宜，則須察乎敵之強弱，強則避之，宜以智取。
弱則攻之，可以力敵。要在速進速退，不使敵人得乘其
隙。所謂〝高低隨時；縱橫因勢〞者是也。

The advancing and retreating must respond to the actual situations in a fight. When you have an advantageous opportunity, advance, and when you are in an urgent position, retreat. This refers to strategy. Naturally, this strategy also includes dodging sideways, up and down movement, and the to and fro of the hands. Timing is very important in the strategy of a fight. Therefore, your Yi must decide quickly, and your actions must be firm, fast, and without hesitation. Your Yi cannot be separated from all of these strategic movements. When the opponent is strong, your strategy is different from when you are fighting against someone who is weak. The last sentence of this section: "High and low following the time (i.e., opportunity), vertical and horizontal following the situation" truly expresses the key to strategy.

The seventh is the body movement must be speedy. In Xingyi Wushu, all of the Five Phases, Six Unifications, Seven Speeds, and Eight Importances rely on the body as the foundation. It is said: "The body is like the bow and the fist is like the arrow." It is again said: "the high level techniques require that the body moves first and the hands and legs all immediately follow and become a real (complete) technique." Therefore, the body movements are the foundation of Xingyiquan. Loose shoulders, lively hips, the entire body can be turned, and the body moves forward at an angle. Should not bow forward and lean backward, lean to the left and tilt to the right. When it is forward, then straight forward, and when retreating then straight backward. Especially must pay attention to the unifica-

tion of the internal and external. The entire body must stick together, upper and lower parts are like one. When moving forward or retreating, it cannot be broken. Then the opportunity cannot be gauged and the opponent cannot achieve his intention. This is why, in addition to the eyes speed, hand speed, etc., you must consider the body's speed precious.

七·身法要疾。形意武術中凡五行、六合、七疾、八要等法,皆以身法為本。譜云:「身如弩弓拳如箭;」又云:「上法須要先上身,手腳齊到方為真。」故身法者,形意拳術之本也。搖膀活胯,週身輾轉,側身而進,不可前俯後仰,左歪右斜。進則直出,退則直落,尤必顧到內外相合,務使其週身團結,上下如一,雖進退不能破散,則庶幾不可捉摸,而敵不得逞,此所以於眼疾、手疾等外,而尤貴乎其身疾也。

The last important factor in winning a battle is the body's movements. The body here means the torso. Since the limbs are attached to the body, if your body does not move fast, even though the limbs are fast the techniques will not be fast and effective. Therefore, the body is the foundation of the hands and legs, and they can move fast only when this foundation is able to move fast.

Jin originates with the legs, is directed by the waist, and manifests in the hands. Therefore, if your waist cannot direct the power generated from the legs quickly, the power will be reduced and ineffective. Finally, the body movement here should also include the internal Qi movement. The Qi is stored at the Lower Dan Tian, and when Jin is emitted, this Qi is led to the limbs to manifest Jin.

The Song of Seven Stars 七星歌

When (Xingyiquan is) used, it must have seven bodies: the head, the shoulders, the elbows, and the hands. (Also) combined with the hips, knees, and feet, and mutually assisting as friends.

用必七體,頭肩肘手,胯膝合腳,相助為友。

The text following this poem in the original document explains that when Xingyiquan is practiced, the linking steppings are used, which are usually practiced in the Linking Sequence. These steppings are called "stepping seven stars (Ta Qi Xing, 踏七星)." When you are practicing the Linking Sequence, in every movement the seven bodies must coordinate with each other. Only then will your entire body act like a unit and the techniques be effective. The seven bodies include: head, two shoulders (and hips), two elbows (and knees), and two hands (and feet).

The Song of Fighting #1 打手歌一

(In) the technique of striking, you must move your body first. It is real only when both your feet and hands arrive (together). The fist is shaped like a cannon and the body bent like a dragon. When you encounter the opponent, it is like your body is on fire.

打法定要先上身，腳手齊到才為真。拳如炮形龍折身，
遇敵好似火燒身。

This again emphasizes that in a fight, the body must move first. Only then can your hands and feet also arrive. When a fist is used to strike, its power is like a cannonball shot from a cannon. When the body moves and stores Jin, it can be flexible like a dragon. When you face your opponent, you are alert and agile, and you look like your body is about to catch fire. When you attack, you are as powerful, active, and dangerous as fire.

When the striking Yi is generated, the head is in the center. When the entire body arrives all together, the opponent cannot defend. The feet are stepping in the center door to occupy the advantageous position. Even if (your opponent) is a fairy, he will have difficulty defending.

頭打起意站中央，渾身齊到人難當。腳踩中門奪地位，
就是神仙亦難防。

This section points out two important things. The first is that the head is suspended when Yi is generated in a fight. Only then will your body be centered and balanced, which allows your entire body to move forward and backward steadily and firmly. The second is that in strategy, you must always catch the opportunity to occupy the "center door" (Zhong Men, 中門), which is right in front of the opponent's chest. If you can occupy this door, you will be able to access the opponent's most vital areas on the front side of his body.

(When) the shoulder is striking for one Yin, you again return with one Yang. Both hands are always hidden in a dark place. Left and right (strikes) all depend on the advantages of postures. Withdrawing and extending (are just) two words, one life will be terminated.

肩打一陰返一陽，兩手只在暗處藏。左右全憑蓋勢取，
縮長二字一命亡。

The shoulder is considered the root of the arms. In the arm, the shoulder is the root, the elbow is the middle section, and the hand is the end section. When there is an Yi for a hand strike, the root section sets up for the strike. This is Yin. When the strike is emitted to the hands and the power is manifested, it is Yang. In this song, it says that when one of your hands is striking (Yang), the other should have already stored the Jin (Yin) for the next strike. You must not let your opponent know what your hands will do. It should be like they are hiding in a dark place. That means your opponent will not be able to figure out the substantial and insubstantial of your strike. These attacks and withdrawals should not be rigid and dead. They should be agile and alive, and correspond to the advantages of the situation.

> *(When) the hands strike, the Yi is on the (opponent's) chest. Their vehemence is like a tiger leaping toward a lamb. (When) you stick firmly and use Li, they should be extended and loose. The two elbows should always (remain) hidden under the armpits.*

> 手打起意在胸膛，其勢好似虎撲羊。沾實用力須展放，
> 兩肘只在脅下藏。

Xingyiquan's strategy focuses on occupying the center door, and the fists are used mainly to strike the opponent's chest area. In order to make the Jin reach to the opponent's body, your Yi must be on the target, otherwise your Yi will not lead your Qi and energize the muscles so that they can manifest the Jin. When you strike, you must use power and speed, like a tiger attacking a lamb. While you are striking, the muscles should be loose and extended. The elbows should always be sunken (or dropped) so that the Jin will be rooted and strong. This will also protect the vital areas under the armpits.

> *(When) the hips are used for striking, left and right should be relaxed and move easily. The exchange of both feet should be natural. (When) moving forward, left or right should have the sword's Jin. When the hands move as the mind wishes, the opponent will be turned over automatically.*

> 胯打陰陽左右便，兩足交換須自然。左右進取宜劍勁，
> 得心應手敵自翻。

The hips connect the body to the legs, which are its root. They are also responsible for the body's movement. In Xingyiquan, the hips are considered to be the root, the knees are the middle section, and the feet are the end section. Therefore, only when these roots move first can the entire body be mobile. When you move, the hips should be relaxed and easy. Whether you move to the left or right, forward or backward, depends upon what is convenient and appropriate. Then, the feet can move naturally as they switch back and forth. When you move, you must move straight forward and backward quickly and firmly, like a sword. You must move directly and without hesitation. When your Yi has made a decision, your hands move in coordination with the legs to easily execute it.

> *(When) knees are used for striking, they can cause death. Two hands feint movement in the upper center. (It is) a marvelous secret and you are advised to practice diligently. Unlimited happiness will be gained from strengthening the body and defeating the opponent.*

> 膝打要害能致命，兩手空幌繞上中。妙訣勸君勤練習，
> 強身勝敵樂無窮。

It is believed that the elbows can be more destructive than the hands, while the knees can be more dangerous than the feet. Because Xingyiquan specializes in short-range fighting, knee strikes are very important. When you intend to use your knees for an attack, you should first move your hands in front of your opponent's upper body. This feint will attract his attention and cause him to raise his defenses, leaving his lower body open to your attack. You must practice this trick until you can convince the opponent that your hands are the real attack as you set up for the knee attack.

(When) the feet step, the Yi must be firm and accurate and not enter the emptiness. The message (i.e., key) relies entirely on the rear leg's kicking. (When) storing your Yi, you should prevent being sensed by your opponent. (When) you start to move, it is like a tornado.

腳踩正意勿落空，消息全在後腳蹬。蓄意須防被敵覺，
起勢好似捲地風。

When your Yi has made a decision, you must be firm and not change your mind. This way your stepping will be firm and accurate and your strategy will not be in vain. The key is that your movement originates with your "kicking off" from your rear leg. You can use this movement to step forward, to retreat, or even to kick. You can also use this movement to suddenly kick. When you retreat, you do the same thing, only now you kick off with the front leg. When you are storing Jin just before you move, you must be careful to act naturally so that your opponent does not feel or sense your preparation. If he does, your technique will not work.

The Song of Fighting #2 打手歌二

(When) the fists are used for striking, the shape of the three sections cannot be seen. If the shape and the shadow can be seen, then (the strike) cannot be said to be proficient. Proficiency comes right after the end of the thought, and does not dally with the thought. The proficiency is (generated) before the Qi and not after the Qi.

拳打三節不見形，如見形影不為能。能在一思進，莫在
一思存。能在一氣先，莫在一氣後。

When you strike, you should not let your opponent feel or sense it, otherwise, it is useless. The key to making the technique proficient is that the strike should be executed immediately right after the Yi has made the decision. If you hesitate and question your decision, your opponent will be able to sense your strategy. In addition, your Yi (thought) must be ahead of the Qi. Only then can your Qi be efficiently led to support the technique. The last sentence means that proficiency is decided before Qi is led, not after. Once the Qi has been led, it is already too late.

(When) the hips are used for striking the middle section, both of them are connected. Yin and Yang mutually combined is hard to obtain. (If) the external hips are like a fish jumping, then (it will be) hard to hide the stepping (i.e., strategy) and change the postures in the internal hips.

胯打中節并相連，陰陽相合得之難。外胯好似魚打挺，
裡胯藏步變勢難。

When your techniques are directed at the opponent's stomach and abdomen, your power is rooted in your hips. In order to make the strike powerful, both hips should be connected (i.e., coordinated with each other), and Yin and Yang should be coordinated. The hip of the rear leg is Yin, and the hip of the front leg is Yang. When both hips are connected and coordinated, their power can be rooted in the ground. However, if the hips are loose and flop around like a fish on the land, then the stepping will not be firm and steady, and your opponent will be able to gauge your stepping strategy.

(When) the knees are striking at the several places, the opponent will not know. (They are) like a fierce tiger escaping from the cage: the body is harmonious when turning, do not stop your movements. Repel left and right clearly and strike as desired.

膝打幾處人不明，好似猛虎出木籠。和身轉著不停式，
左右明撥任意行。

There are only a few places you can effectively attack with the knees: the abdomen, the groin, and the thighs. However, if executed correctly, it is very hard for the opponent to tell which target you are going to attack. Once you start your strike, you are just like a fierce tiger escaping from a tiny cage. Your body can move or turn easily and continuously to set up an opportunity for your strike, and you can choose any target you wish.

When the hips and the tail are used for striking, movement up and down cannot be seen. It is like a fierce tiger entering and leaving his cave.

臀尾打，起落不見形，好似猛虎坐臥出洞中。

When you are crouching just before an attack, you accumulate postural power and Qi in your lower body. This is done subtly so that the opponent cannot see it. It is like a tiger carefully coming out of his cave in a crouch, drawing in his body and preparing to pounce on his prey.

The Seven Followings of Xingyiquan 形意拳七順

The shoulders should urge (i.e., push) the elbows, and the elbows should not oppose the shoulders. The elbows should urge the hands, and the hands should not oppose the elbows. The hands should urge the fingers, and the fingers should not oppose the hands. The waist should urge the hips, and the hips should not oppose the waist. The hips should urge the knees, and the knees should not oppose the hips. The knees should urge the feet, and the feet should not oppose the knees. The head should urge the body, and the body should not oppose the head. Xin and Qi are steady, Yin and Yang mutually unify. The top and the bottom are mutually connected, internal and external are combined like one. This is called the seven followings.

肩要催肘，而肘不逆肩。肘要催手，而手不逆肘。手要催指，而指不逆手。腰要催胯，而胯不逆腰。胯要催膝，而膝不逆胯。膝要催足，而足不逆膝。首要催身，而身不逆首。心氣穩定，陰陽相合，上下相連，內外如一，此之謂七順。

When you emit Jin, your mind generates the idea, and your body should carry it out without any kind of resistance. The movement starts in the body and extends out simultaneously through the arms and legs. As the force is transmitted out the limbs, it should move smoothly and uniformly. Each part of the body accepts the force from the part of the body behind it, and transmits it to the next part. Nothing should hinder this free flow of force. Once your mind decides to act, it should not hesitate or question the decision. If your resolve is steady, the Qi will be too. Yin and Yang must be unified, which means that a movement in one direction should be balanced with a simultaneous movement in the opposite direction.

This document explains that in the three sections, the root section usually generates the power, the middle section transmits and directs the power, and the end section manifests the power. Each section pushes the next one until the Jin is out. If the passage of Jin through the body is smooth and without any resistance, then the three sections can be connected as a unit. There are many ways to divide the body into threes, and each of these sections should be connected together as one. In addition, the internal and the external must also be combined, otherwise you could not call Xingyiquan an internal martial art.

The Eight Postures of Xingyiquan 形意拳八勢

There are eight important points in the postures of Xingyiquan. The first is Ding (press), the second is Ti (hold up), the third is Kou (arc/grab), the fourth is Yuan (round), the fifth is Bao (embrace), the sixth is Chui (drop), the seventh is Heng (sideways) and Shun (smoothness) must be known (i.e., understood) clearly, and the eighth is raising up for Zuan (drill) and down for Fan (turn over) must be clearly distinguished.

形意拳之姿勢，其重要之點有八：一曰頂，二曰提，三曰扣，四曰圓，五曰抱，六曰垂，七橫順須知情，八起鑽落翻須分明。

The eight important postures are discussed in two different sources. They differ on three postures, and they both have their unique point of view.

Ding (press) means the head is pressing upward, the tongue is pressing upward to the roof of the mouth, and the hands are pressing forward. Ti (hold up) means the tailbone (Weilu) is lifting up and the anus is held up internally. Kou (arc/grab) means the chest must be arced, the back of the hands must be arced, and the bottom of the feet must be arced downward. Yuan (round) means the back must be round, the tiger's mouth (between the thumb and index finger) must be half-round, the arms and the shoulders must be like the early moon. When the hands and the wrists are pressing forward, they must also be like the early moon. When the legs are bent, they are like the early moon. Bao (embrace) means the (Lower) Dan Tian must be embraced, the heart must be embraced, the arms and shoulders must be embraced. Chui (drop) means the Qi is dropped to the (Lower) Dan Tian, the shoulders are dropped, and the elbow tips are dropped.

頂者，頭往上頂，舌尖頂上齶，手往外頂是也。提者，
尾閭上提，穀道內提是也。扣者，胸脯要扣，手背要扣，
腳面要往下扣是也。圓者，脊背要圓，虎口要半圓，胳
膊要月芽形，手腕外頂要月芽形，腿曲連灣要月芽形是
也。抱者，丹田要抱，心中要抱，胳膊要抱是也。垂者，
氣垂丹田，膀尖下垂，肘尖下垂是也。

When the head presses upward, you are raising your spirit of vitality. Your head should feel like it is suspended, and you should remain relaxed. It is your Yi which presses your head upward, and when this is done correctly your physical body will become light as if it were suspended from above. The tongue must also press upward to touch the roof of the mouth in order to connect the Yin Conception (Ren Mai, 任脈) and Yang Governing Vessels (Du Mai, 督脈). Even though the tongue is pressed up, it remains relaxed. If the tongue is tensed, then the Qi will be stagnant there. Next, the hands must be pressed forward. Only when your Yi is pressing forward will it be ahead of the Qi, so that it can lead the Qi.

Although this poem uses the term "tailbone," it in fact means the anus and the Huiyin (Co-1)(會陰) cavity. The Huiyin cavity is located between the anus and the genitals (Figure 2-2). When the anus and the Huiyin cavity are lifted, the tailbone will also naturally be lifted. In Qigong practice, the Huiyin is considered one of the "tricky gates" which can control Kan (坎)(Water) and Li (離)(Fire) for Yin and Yang adjustment. Holding up and relaxing the Huiyin cavity and the anus are the keys to this adjustment. For more information, please refer to Dr. Yang's book *The Root of Chinese Qigong.*

The third key posture is arcing (Kou, 扣). This includes the arcing of the chest, the back of the hands, and the bottom of the feet. When the chest is arced, the lungs will be relaxed and the Jin can be stored in the arcing posture. When the hands are arced, Qi can be gathered in the palms, and Jin can be manifested strongly. When the bottom of the feet are arced slightly, they will be relaxed and the Qi will be able to communicate with the ground and build up a firm root.

The back is round, which actually means that the chest is arced. When the tiger mouth areas of the hands are half round, the Qi can be strongly spread out to the palms and the Jin can be manifested efficiently. The arms and the shoulders are round in order to have the best posture for storing Jin. When the hands are used to press forward, the back of the wrists should not be 90 degrees. They should be slightly curved. Consequently the wrist areas will not be tensed and the Qi can be transported easily through them. When the legs are slightly bent, the posture is firm and the root can be strong.

When you have the feeling that the Lower Dan Tian area is embraced, the Qi can be gathered there. When the heart is embraced, your emotional mind will have a center and will not be distracted by your opponent. When the arms and the shoulders are embraced, the Jin can be effectively stored and the vital areas in the chest can be well-protected.

The next key is that the Qi must be sunk to the Lower Dan Tian. Only then can the Qi be full and abundant in the Lower Dan Tian and the mind be clear. It is like when you let muddy water sit quietly for a while, and the mud settles to the bottom leaving the water on top clear. Next, the shoulders and the elbows must drop so that they will be able to relax and the Jin can be stored efficiently. In addition, dropping the shoulders and elbows protects the vital areas, especially the armpits.

> *Heng (sideways) means to rise and Shun (smoothness) means to descend. Raise means to Zuan (drill upwards) and descend means to Fan (turn over). Raising is the beginning of Heng (sideways), and Zuan (drill) is the end of Heng. Descending is the beginning of Shun (smoothness), and Fan (turn over) is the end of smoothness. The hands rise for Zuan (drill) and the hand descend for Fan (turn over). The feet rise for Zuan (drill) and descend for Fan (turn over). Raising is going and descending is striking. When it is raised, it is for striking, when it is descending it is also for striking. It does not matter how you rise and fall, Zuan (drill) and Fan (turn over), to or fro, in all the elbows must not leave the place under the armpits, the hands do not leave the heart (mind), these are the postures which should be paid attention to when practicing Xingyiquan.*

横者，起也。順者，落也。起者，鑽也。落者，翻也。
起為橫之始，鑽為橫之終。落為順之始，翻為順之終。
手起而鑽，手落而翻。足起而鑽，足落而翻。起是去，
落是打。起亦打，落亦打。勿論如何起落鑽翻往來，總
要肘不離脅，手不離心，此形意拳之所宜注意之姿勢也。

The last two key postures discuss attacking strategy and the movements. The first key movement includes Heng (橫) and Shun (順) and the second movement includes Zuan (鑽) and Fan (翻). Heng in Chinese has the meaning of forcing one's way in by pushing obstacles aside. It is an aggressive movement sideward and diagonally. In Xingyiquan, the Heng motion is used together with Zuan (drill). In fact, although Heng and Zuan are used to clear the way for further strikes, very often when there is no obstacle to be cleared they can be used directly as an attack.

However, when there is an obstacle in the way you clear it out with Heng and Zuan, then you follow with the techniques of Shun and Fan. Shun in Chinese means to follow smoothly, and here it means that after you have cleared the way you strike downward diagonally to the opponent's body. Once you have cleared the obstacles which stop you from entering a door, you are then able to enter smoothly. In Xingyiquan, this motion is very often used together with Fan. Fan means to turn over. When you use Shun to reach the opponent's body, you are also turning your limbs to generate the drilling and penetrating power. These two key postures also apply to the legs.

The Song of the Eight Postures 八字歌訣

The eight words (i.e., key postures), are Ding (press), Kou (arc/grab), Yuan (round), Min (acute), Bao (embrace), Chui (drop), Qu (bend), and Ting (thrust). When the stance and the forms of the fists are formed, all these eight words must have been observed. Therefore, (you are) able to store the Li and build up the Qi. (This) makes it possible that the person who is my enemy does not know how to deal with it. These are the special characteristics of the Five Phases. Within these eight words, there are again three classifications in each one of them.

八字者，頂、扣、圓、敏、抱、垂、曲、挺是也。庄法
及拳式站定時，此八字須具備焉。所以蓄力養氣，使敵
我者，無所措使。斯亦五行拳所持有者也。而八字者，
又各有三種焉。

Three of these eight key postures are different from those of the previous document. That is because they are a different master's explanation of his understanding of the postures. Understanding both documents will increase the depth of your understanding of the art.

The first is the "three pressed" (San Ding). What are the three pressings? The head is pressing upward, seeming like it is going to thrust into the sky. The head is the master of the entire body. When the head is pressed, then the three gates on the back can be passed through easily and the kidneys' Qi can therefore reach upward to the Ni Wan (i.e., dust pill) for the nourishment of the human nature. (When) the hands are pressing outward, they have the achievement of pushing a mountain. Then the Qi can be threaded and reach to the entire body, and the Li can reach to the four limbs. (When) the tongue is pressing upward, (you) have the ability to roar like a lion and swallow an elephant. (This) makes it possible to lead the rising kidney Qi downward to return to the (Lower) Dan Tian and solidify the lifeforce. These are called "San Ding."

一曰三頂。三頂者何？頭向上頂，有衝天之雄。頭為週
身之主，上頂則後三關易通，腎氣因之上達泥丸以養性。
手掌外頂，有推山之功，則氣貫週身，力達四肢。舌上
頂，有吼獅吞象之容，能導上升之腎氣，下行歸入丹田
以固命。是謂之三頂。

The key word "press" (Ding, 頂) has three parts. The first one is that the head is pressing upward. When you do this, the head is upright and suspended. The spirit can be raised, and, because your posture is correct, the Qi will be able to pass through the three "gates" (San Guan, 三關) on the back of your body where the Qi may have difficulty getting through. These three gates are the Tailbone (Weilu, 尾閭), Squeeze Spine (Jiaji, 夾脊), and the Jade Pillow (Yuzhen, 玉枕). For a detailed discussion of these three gates, consult *The Root of Chinese Qigong* and *Qigong—Secret of Youth* by Dr. Yang. "Ni Wan" (泥丸) is the Qigong term for the brain. According to Chinese Qigong theory, Original Qi (Yuan Qi, 元氣) comes from the conversion of Original Essence (Yuan Jing, 元精), which resides in the kidneys. When the Qi can pass smoothly through the three gates, the Original Qi will be able to reach the brain and nourish it.

The second press is the hands pressing. The hands should always have the feeling that they are pressing forward. This leads Qi to your hands, and also energizes your whole body. When the hands are used for pressing or punching, their power should be so strong that they could push a mountain. When you have the Yi of pushing on your hands, then your Yi will also be able to lead the Qi to the extremities and energize the entire body.

The third press is the tongue pressing. The tongue should press upward and touch the roof of the mouth. This connects the Conception and Governing Vessels and lets the Qi flow smoothly. This pressing makes it possible for the Qi to be sunk to the Lower Dan Tian (the residence of Original Qi) so that you can conserve your Original Qi and keep your body strong.

> *The second is the three arc/grabs (San Kou). What are the three arcings? Two shoulders must be arcing, then the front of the chest is wide with space. Qi and Li will (therefore) reach the elbows. The back of the hands and the top of the feet must be arcing, then Qi and Li will reach the hands and make the stance firm and Li strong. The teeth must be closed, then the tendons and bones are strongly controlled. These are called "San Kou" (three arc/grabs).*

二曰三扣。三扣者何？兩肩要扣，則前胸空闊，氣力到
肘。手背、足背要扣，則氣力到手，庄步力厚。牙齒要
扣，則筋骨緊縮。是謂之三扣。

The second important posture is arcing. There are three places which are arced. The first place is the shoulders, which should be arced forward. This opens and relaxes your chest and eases your breathing. In addition, since the shoulders are the root of the arms, the arcing of the shoulders provides firm support for the elbows.

The second place that should arc is the back of the hands and the back of the feet. Arcing strengthens the hands for grabbing, and allows the feet to make firm contact with the ground (to "grab" it) so that you can build up a strong root. The third place is the teeth, which must be closed tight. (The Chinese word "Kou" also has this meaning.) This makes it possible for the Qi to reach to the tendons and bones and make them strong.

> *The third is three rounds (San Yuan). What are the three rounds? The back must be round, (then) its Li is able to destroy the (opponent's) body, and the tailbone will be centered and upright. (In this case), the spirit of vitality will be able to reach the top (of the head). The chest must be round, then the Li on the two elbows is complete. The heart cave (i.e., solar plexus) arcs slightly in, the breathing will be unhindered and smooth. The Tiger's Mouth must be round, the bravery and fierceness can be stimulated, then the hands have embracing power. These are called "San Yuan" (the three rounds).*

三曰三圓。三圓者何？脊背要圓，其力催身，則尾閭中正，精神貫頂。前胸要圓，兩肘力全，心窩微收，呼吸通順。虎口要圓，勇猛外宣，則心有裹抱力。是謂之三圓。

Three places in the posture are round. The first two are the back and the chest. The thoracic vertebrae should be slightly curved, which will also round the shoulders forward in a bear-like posture. The chest is also relaxed and rounded inward. When the back, chest, and shoulders are rounded, power from the shoulders will be able to connect to the waist and be directed to the root of the body. Only then will your entire body act as a unit and connect to the ground. Naturally, when you arc your back you should still keep your body upright and your head suspended. When you have the posture right, the solar plexus area will be loose and the lungs will be able to move easily and smoothly.

The third place that should be round is the Tiger's Mouth (Hu Kou, 虎口), which is the martial arts term for the place between the thumb and the index finger. When this area is round, the Qi is able to reach to the finger tips and strengthen your grabbing power.

> *The fourth is the three acutes (San Min). What are the three acutes? The Xin (emotional mind) must be acute, like an angry fox catching a rat. Then (you) can change (your strategy) to correspond to the situation. The eyes must be acute, like a hungry eagle seizing a rabbit. (Then you) will be able to predict the proper opportunity. The hands must be acute, like a hungry tiger catching a lamb. (Then you) will be able to control the opponent first. These are called "San Min" (the three acutes).*

四曰三敏。三敏者何？心要敏，如怒狸攫鼠，則能隨機應變。眼要敏，如饑鷹之捉兔，能預視察機宜。手要敏，如捕羊之餓虎，能先發制人。是謂之三敏。

The Chinese word "Min" (敏) means many things. It can mean "smart," "alert," "fast action," "acute reaction," and "sensitive feeling." The first acute is the emotional mind (Xin). When the eyes pass information to the mind, it is the emotional mind which receives it first, then the wisdom mind makes its judgement. When the emotional mind is acute, you will be alert and will be able to keep your spirit high. Only then will you be able to feel or sense the situation appropriately and find opportunities.

The second acute is the eyes. The eyes provide your first contact with the opponent. When the eyes are sharp, they are able to pass accurate information to the mind. The third acute is the hands. Once the mind has made its decision, the hands must react quickly. Only then will your entire body be agile and your responses alive.

> *The fifth is the three embraces (San Bao). What are the three embracings? The (Lower) Dan Tian must be embraced, (so) the Qi will not exit outward. (Then) when attacking the opponent, (the power) will be accurate. The Xin and Qi must be embraced. (Then) there is a master when encountering the opponent which enables (your mind to be) steady when there is a sudden (strategy) change (by your opponent). Two (sides of) the ribs must be embraced. (Then) releasing and withdrawing will have order and there is no danger when encountering the opponent. These are called "San Bao" (the three embraces).*

> 五曰三抱。三抱者何？丹田要抱，氣不外散，擊敵必準。
> 心氣要抱，遇敵有主，臨變不變。兩肋要抱，出入不亂，
> 遇敵無險。是謂之三抱。

The word "Bao" (抱) includes several different feelings. Bao can be translated as embrace, hold together, stick together, enfold, harbor, or cherish. The first embrace is that the mind must remain at the Lower Dan Tian. This keeps the Qi at its residence so that it can be strong and abundant. Only then, when you store your Jin, will you have plenty of Qi to make the techniques fast and sharp.

The second embrace is that the emotional mind and the Qi must stick together. Since Qi is led by your Yi, this also implies that your Xin and Yi must be together. In other words, when the Xin is touched by something, the Yi immediately makes a judgement and the Qi is led automatically. When you embrace your Xin, Qi, and Yi, your mind will have a center and will not be confused. Even if there is a sudden change in the situation, you will not be alarmed or afraid. The third embrace is that your elbows must sink and be held in (embrace the ribs). This gives your hands a firm root in attack and defense, and will also protect your armpits.

> *The sixth is the three drops (San Chui). What are the three drops? Qi must be dropped (i.e., sunk), the Qi is sunk to the (Lower) Dan Tian and the body is steady like a mountain. The two shoulders must be dropped, then the shoulders are extended and agile (and) able to urge the elbows to move forward. The two elbows must be dropped, then the two forearms are rounded automatically, (and) able to strengthen the flanks. These are called "San Chui" (the three drops).*

六曰三垂。三垂者何？氣垂則氣降丹田，身穩如山。兩
肩下垂，則臂長而活，肩催肘前。兩肘下垂，則兩肱自
圓，能固兩脅。是謂之三垂。

"Chui" (垂) means to drop, fall, sink, or bow. The first drop is that the Qi must be sunk to the Lower Dan Tian, then it will always be kept at its center. This will make the body rooted and steady like a mountain, and your power will have a firm energy source. The second drop is the shoulders. This connects the shoulders to the body so that the Jin manifested in the arms will have a root and foundation. For the same reason, the elbows must be sunken so that they are connected firmly to the shoulders. This will also protect your armpits.

The seventh is the three bends (San Qu). What are the three bends? The two fore-arms should be bent, bow-shape like the half moon, then the Li is abundant. The two knees should be bent, bent like the half moon, then Li is thick. The two wrists should be bent, curved like the half moon, then Li is gathered. All of these (joints) are adapted to extending and withdrawing as desired and the Jin can be applied without stopping. These are called "San Qu" (the three bends).

七曰三曲。三曲者何？兩肱宜曲，弓如半月，則力富。
兩膝宜曲，彎如半月，則力厚。手腕宜曲，曲如半月，
則力湊。皆取其伸縮自如，用勁不斷之意。是謂之三曲。

A curve or bend is the key to storing Jin in the postures. It is like a bow which is bent and ready to shoot an arrow. This "curve" or "bend" (Qu, 曲) is different from "round" (Yuan, 圓). When you curve or bend a joint you are storing Jin, just like a bent bow stores energy. "Round" refers to curving or arcing your posture to smooth the Qi circulation and to neutralize the opponent's Jin. There are three places in the body where the Jin can be stored in Xingyiquan. They are the arms, the wrists, and the legs. If you are able to bend them smoothly and naturally, you will be able to extend them or bend them without effort. In this case, the Jin can be stored and emitted as you wish.

The eighth is the three thrusts (San Ting). What are the three thrusts? The neck and the head thrust upward, then the head area is straight and (lifting) upward and the spirit of vitality can reach the top. The spine bones and the waist must be thrust up, then Li can reach the four extremities, (and) the Qi can be like a drum in the entire body. Both knees are thrust out (i.e., strong and firm), then the Qi is peaceful and the Shen is harmonious, like a tree having a firm root.

八曰三挺。三挺者何？頸項挺，則頭部正直，精氣貫頂。
脊骨要挺，則力達四梢，氣鼓全身。膝蓋挺，則氣恬神
怡，如樹生根。

"Ting" (挺) in Chinese has the meaning of standing upright, rigid, firm and strong, straightened, and thrusting out. When the neck and head are thrust up or straightened, the head will be suspended and the spirit of vitality can be raised. Second, the spine and the waist must also be thrust up and straightened, then the body will be able to keep its center and balance. Only when your body is centered will your power be able to reach the four limbs efficiently. In addition, through correct body posture, the Qi stored in the Lower Dan Tian can be full and abundant. Third, the knees must be firm and strong to build up a firm root and to be able to generate the Jin for fighting. It is said: "Jin is generated in the legs, directed by the waist, and manifested in the hands." Only when you have a firm root will your mind be able to be steady, the spirit harmonious, and the Qi transported without interruption.

The Eight Important Points #1 形意拳八要一

(When) the Xin (emotional mind) is steady, the Shen (spirit) is calm. The Shen is calm, the Xin is peaceful. The Xin is peaceful, then it is quiet and clean. It is quiet and clean, then nothing exists. When nothing exists, the Qi will be transported (smoothly). When Qi is transported smoothly, then the imagination disappears. When the imagination disappears, then the feeling (i.e., sensing) is clear. When the feeling is clear, then the Shen and Qi are mutually connected. In this case, millions of Qis return to their roots.

心定，神寧；神寧，心安；心安，清靜；清靜，無物；
無物，氣行；氣行，絕象；絕象，覺明；覺明，則神氣
相通，萬物歸根矣。

When Xin is not steady, the spirit will be disturbed, but when the spirit is able to be calm, the Xin can be directed into a peaceful state. Only when your emotional mind is peaceful, quiet, and free from miscellaneous thoughts will your spirit be able to reach the Wuji state (無極)(i.e., the state of emptiness). In this quiet state your mind rests in emptiness or "nothingness," and it feels as if the physical body had disappeared. Your entire body is then transparent to the Qi, which can flow freely and without obstruction. Then your imagination will not play tricks on you and distract you, and your feelings (sensory perception) will be neutral and clear. Consequently, the spirit and Qi can be united as one and you can penetrate to the root of things. You can see from this that the eight important points are: Xin Ding (心定)(steady emotional mind), Shen Ning (神寧)(calm spirit), Xin An (心安) (peaceful emotional mind), Qing Jing (清靜)(cleanness), Wu Wu (無物)(nothingness), Qi Xing (氣行)(Qi transportation), Jue Xiang (絕象)(stop imagination), and Jue Ming (覺明)(clear feeling).

The Eight Important Points #2 形意拳八要二

What are the eight important points? First, inside must be lifted. Second, the three centers must be together. Third, the three Yis must be linked together. Fourth, the Five Phases must be smooth. Fifth, the four extremities must be uniform. Sixth, the Xin must be leisurely. Seventh, the three tips must face each other. Eighth, the eyes must be venomous.

八要者何？一‧內心要提；二‧三心要并；三‧三意要
連；四‧五行要順；五‧四梢要齊；六‧心要暇；七‧
三尖要對；八‧眼要壽也。

You can see that the eight important points listed in this document are not the same as those in the previous document. This document goes on to explain them.

"Inside must be held up (Ti)" means tightening up the grain path (i.e., anus) to raise up the Qi and enable it to gather at the (Lower) Dan Tian. Again, make the Qi gathered at the (Lower) Dan Tian (move) through the spine back (thoracic vertebrae) and reach the brain directly. Transport (Qi) in a cycle to and fro so that the circulation has no end. This is what is called "tightening the grain path and holding up internally."

內要提者，緊撮穀道，提其氣使上聚於丹田，復使聚於
丹田之氣，由背脊而直達於腦頂，週流往返，循環無端，
即所謂〝緊撮穀道內中提〞也。

The Chinese word "Ti" (提) means to hold up. Very often it is translated as lift or raise, however, in Chinese Qigong "hold up" is more accurate. In order to do the "hold up" posture, you must slightly tighten up the anus area. When you are holding up a bucket of water you don't need to lift or raise it. When you lift or raise the bucket, the muscles must be tensed, and this will stagnate the Qi circulation. However, if you simply hold it up, although the muscles are slightly tensed, the Yi is stronger than the actual physical activity and the muscles may remain relaxed and not inhibit the smooth circulation of Qi. "Ti" is a key word in Qigong and internal martial arts. With Ti, the Qi can be raised upward from the bottom of the feet to the Lower Dan Tian, and then follow the spine upward to nourish the brain. The Ti word is the key to the Kan (坎)(Water) and Li (離)(Fire) adjustment of the body's Yin and Yang. When you are practicing the Ti word, the Huiyin (Co-1)(會陰)(cavity between the groin and anus) and the anus should be held up internally. Remember, the Yi is more important than the physical tensing. When you do this properly, the Qi can be led upward to complete the Fire path or Water path Qi circulation. This subject is discussed more thoroughly in several of Dr. Yang's books.

"Three centers must be together" means the center of the head is led downward, the centers of the feet are led upward, and the centers of the hands move to and fro. These three places enable the Qi to gather in one place. Because if the center of the head is not led downward, then the Qi on the top cannot be moved down to the (Lower) Dan Tian. If the centers of the feet are not directed upward, then

the lower Qi cannot be collected at the (Lower) Dan Tian. If the centers of the hands are not moving to and fro, then the external Qi cannot be withdrawn to the (Lower) Dan Tian. Therefore, the three centers must be together so Qi can be returned to one (place).

三心要并者，頂心往下，腳心往上，手心往回也。三者
所以使氣會於一處。蓋頂心不往下，則上氣不能入於丹
田；腳心不往上，則下氣不能收於丹田；手心不往回，
則外氣不能收於丹田。故必三心一并，而氣始可歸於一
也。

The "one place" here means the Lower Dan Tian, which is the center and the residence of Qi. When Jin is emitted, the Qi stored in the Lower Dan Tian is led to the limbs, and when Jin is stored, the Qi in the body is led to the Lower Dan Tian. Therefore, when you are storing Jin and inhaling, the Qi in the head must be led downward, the Qi in the bottoms of the feet must be led upward, and the Qi in the hands must be led inward to the Lower Dan Tian. When you exhale for Jin manifestation, you are leading the Qi to the head for raising up your spirit, to the legs to firm your root, and to the hands to emit the Jin. These three flows of Qi all use the Lower Dan Tian as the gathering place. Only when the Qi has its controlling center (residence) will the Qi circulating in the body have a root and the techniques be skillful and powerful.

"The three Yis must be linked together" means the Xin Yi, Qi Yi, and the Li Yi must be connected into one. This is what is called "the three internal connections." Among these three, the Xin is the planner, the Qi is the marshal, and the Li is the generals and soldiers. Because if the Qi is not full, then Li will not be sufficient. Although the Xin has the plan, it is still in vain (i.e., empty). Therefore, when the Qi and Yi are trained well, then the marshal is able to use Yi to control Li and correspond internally with the Xin Yi. (In) all the connections of these three Yis, the Qi must especially be the first concern.

三意要連者，心意、氣意、力意，三者連而為一，即所
謂內三合也。此三者以心為謀主，氣為元帥，力為將士。
蓋氣不充，則力不足，心雖有謀，亦無所用。故氣意練
好，而後可以外帥力意，內應心意；而三意之連，尤當
以氣為先務也。

The three Yis here mean the Yi which control the Xin, the Yi which directs and leads the Qi, and the Yi which conducts the Li. If you observe yourself carefully, you will see that the three Yis cannot be separated. First, you must have a Xin generated from your feelings (sensory perceptions). The idea from this Xin is then judged and modified by the Yi, and the course of action is decided. Once this decision is made, the Yi leads the Qi and energizes the appropriate muscles. The Yi still has to conduct the energized muscles to execute the decision correctly. You can see that Xin and Yi do the planning, and Qi is the marshal which activates the muscles and generates Li. The Li is the soldiers which carry out the action.

"The Five Phases must be smooth" means the external Five Phases, which are the five fists. They are Pi, Beng, Pao, Zuan, and Heng. The internal Five Phases are the internal viscera, and are the heart, liver, spleen, lungs, and kidneys. For the five fists in the external Five Phases, their variations and applications all follow their methods. Then (they) repeat with the patterns and bend with rules. When Qi and Li arrive, the posture follows. When the posture arrives, then Qi and Li will be focused. When Qi and Li are full, then the postures are useful. When the postures are trained, the Qi and Li will be increased. Therefore, "the Five Phases must be smooth" means the Qi must be smooth.

五行要順者，外五行為五拳，即劈、弸、炮、鑽、橫是也。內五行為五臟，即心、肝、脾、肺、腎是也。外五行之五拳，變化應用，各順其序，則周中規，折中矩，氣力之所到，而架勢即隨之。架勢之所至，而氣力即注之。氣力充，則架勢為有用，架勢練而氣力乃愈增。故五行要順者，即所以順氣也。

The "Five Phases must be smooth" means the Qi circulating in the internal Five Phases (heart, liver, spleen, lungs, and kidneys) must be smooth, then the Qi led to the external Five Phases (Pi, Beng, Pao, Zuan, and Heng) will be full and abundant. In this case, the external Five Phases will act as they are supposed to and the moving pattern will be correct, and the internal and external phases can be unified. Only under this orderly coordination of the two will the variations and applications follow the correct patterns. It is only under this conditions that the Qi and Li can be unified and strong. All of this comes about only if you practice until the Qi and Li immediately arrive whenever you do a posture.

"Four extremities must be uniform" means the tongue must be pressed upward, the teeth must touch (tightly), the fingers and the toes must arc, the pores must be closed. Because when the tongue is pressing upward to touch the roof of the mouth, then the liquid saliva flows upward and the Qi and blood circulate smoothly. When the teeth are closed tightly, then the Qi will thread to the bone marrow. When the fingers and the toes arc internally, then Qi will flow to the tendons. When the pores are closed tightly, then the entire body's Qi will gather and be strong. What is called "uniform" means in every movement the pressing of the tongue, the touching of the teeth, the arcing of the fingers and toes, the closing of the pores must be together and uniform according to the (correct) methods. There is no distinguishing between first and second, late or fast. That is because of all these four, if there is one missing, then the Qi will disperse and Li will be stagnant. Then you cannot talk about techniques.

四梢要齊者，舌要頂，齒要扣，手指、腳趾要扣，毛孔要緊也。夫舌頂上嗉，則津液上注，氣血流通；兩齒緊扣，則氣貫於骨髓；手指、腳趾內扣，則氣注於筋；毛孔緊，則周身之氣聚而堅。齊之云者，即每一作勢時，舌之頂，齒之扣，手腳趾之扣，毛孔之緊，一齊如法，為之無先後遲速之分。蓋以四者如有一缺點，即氣散而力息，便不足以言枝也。

As mentioned before, the tongue is the extremity of the muscles, the teeth are the extremities of the bones, the nails are the extremities of the tendons, and the hair is the extremity of the blood. In order to fill up the Qi and make it abundant, the Qi must be able to reach the ends of these four extremities. Only then can the Qi reach everywhere in the body and energize the entire physical body to its maximum for fighting. That these four extremities must be uniform means that the Qi must be able to reach all four at the same time, and none is stronger than the others. The Qi must be manifested at these four extremities uniformly.

"The Xin must be leisurely" means that when you train, the Xin should not be alarmed and hasty. Because when alarmed, then (you) have the Yi of fright and fear. When (you are) hasty, then you have the Yi of fast and abrupt. When (you are) frightened, then the Qi must be weak; and when (you are) fast and abrupt, then (your) Qi must be disordered. If (your Qi is) weak and disordered, then (the movements of) hands and feet are not manageable. If (you have) not reached the achievement from daily practice, then (you are) empty internally, and when (you) encounter the event, you will be scared and withdrawing. (In this case), there is no one, when he faces the opponent, who is not scared and hasty. Therefore, the Xin must be leisurely. In fact, this corresponds with the Qi externally and internally.

心要暇者，練時心中不慌不忙之謂也。夫慌有恐懼之意，
忙則有急遽之意。一恐懼則氣必餒，一急遽則氣必亂。
餒亂之時，則手足無所措矣。若平日無練習之功，則心
中虧虛，遇事怯縮，遇敵未有不恐懼，不急遽者；故心
要暇，實與練氣相表裡也。

You already know that your Qi is controlled by your Yi. However, if your Yi is not able to regulate your Xin due to fear or haste, then this Yi will not be able to lead and manage the Qi in an effective way. This means that all of your techniques will lose their efficient Qi supply and become ineffective. Therefore, your Xin must be leisurely. You must be firmly confident in yourself so that your Xin will be leisurely and not fearful and hasty. Leisurely here means that you have plenty of time and ability to handle the situation.

"The three tips must face each other" means the tips of the nose, hands, and feet match each other. When the tips of the hands do not match with the tip of the nose and lean to the left, then beware of a technique from the right and beware of the opening. If it is leaning to the right, then beware of a technique from the left and worry about the opening. When the hands and feet, the feet and the nose do not match, its disadvantage is the same. Furthermore, if the three of them are out of alignment too much, then the entire body's power will not be uniform and not be able to stick together like one. Then Qi will be random and disordered. (In this case), though the center of the head is directed downward, the Qi cannot be led downward easily, though the centers of the feet are directed upward, the Qi cannot be gathered upward easily, and though the centers of the hands move to and fro, the Qi cannot be withdrawn (i.e., condensed) easily. This is the natural principle. Therefore, if the three tips are not aligned, it is really an obstruction to training Qi.

三尖要對者，鼻尖、手尖、腳尖相對也。夫手尖不對鼻
尖，偏於左，則右邊顧法空虛。偏於右，則左邊顧法空
虛。手與腳，腳與鼻不對，其弊亦同。且三者如偏斜過
甚，則周身用力不均，必不能團結如一，而氣因之散漫。
頂心雖往下，而氣不易下行；腳心雖往上，而氣不易上
收；手心雖往回，而氣不易內縮；此自然之理也。故三
尖不對，實與練氣有大妨礙也。

This section talks about the center and balance of posture. If you want your Qi led downward from the head and upward from the feet effectively, the body must be centered and balanced. Only then can your judgement be neutral, your head suspended, your feet rooted, and your body not exposed to an opponent's attack because of a defective posture.

Furthermore, when the body is centered and balanced, the Qi in the center of the hands can be led inward efficiently and the Qi in the Lower Dan Tian can be again directed to the centers of the palms. In order to do this, the three tips must be aligned. These three tips are the tips of the hands, nose, and feet.

"The eyes must be venomous (Du)" means the eyes are acute, sharp, and stern, with a mean and serious look. (Your) original Qi must be full and abundant in order to have these. Therefore, when practicing fist techniques (i.e., martial arts), it is no more than training Qi and Li. Training Li is able to strengthen the body, and training Qi is able to enhance the spirit of vitality. Those whose Gongfu is deep are able to gather (the Qi) at the (Lower) Dan Tian, the five internal organs are comfortable and expanded. Then these people's spirit of vitality must be agile and alive, the brain power must be abundant, two ears, eyes, mouth, and nose organs must be able to function completely. Especially, the eyes must be spiritually enlightened and shining onto others. This is what is called "venomous."

眼要毒者，謂目光銳敏而有威也。毒字即寓有威嚴疾敏
之意，非元氣充盈者，不能有此。蓋習拳術不外乎練氣、
練力。練力可以健身體，練氣可以長精神。功夫深者，
能丹田凝聚，五臟舒展。此人之精神必靈活，腦力必充
足，兩耳口鼻等官，必能各盡其用，而目尤必神采奕奕，
光芒射人，是即所謂毒矣。

"Du" (毒) in Chinese has the meanings of poisonous, noxious, venomous, malicious, and spiteful. When this word is used in a fight, it means the spirit is acute, which is shown in the eyes, and the emotions are aggressive, which reflects from the heart to the eyes. When you are in this fighting spirit, the Qi can be full and the movement can be fast and agile. The eyes are where a person's internal feelings and spirit can be shown externally. If you are able to manifest this spirit, you will frighten the opponent and make him lose his confidence. If before the physical fight, you have won spiritually, then there is no doubt about the final victory. The best fight is the fight with no fighting. This means that if you have a spirit which can make an opponent understand that he has no chance to win, then very often you can avoid an actual, physical fight.

The Nine Songs of Xingyiquan 形意拳九歌

Body: Bowing forward and leaning backward, the Jin from postures cannot be strong. Inclining to the left and leaning to the right, all of these are the sickness (i.e., mistakes) of the body (posture). (The body should be) straight but like leaning, leaning but like straight.

身：前俯後仰，其勢不勁。左側右猗，皆身之病。正而
似斜，斜而似正。

This first song is about the body. The body posture should be centered and balanced. That means you should not lean in any direction. The last sentence sounds like a contradiction. However, according to the feeling of the Chinese, it means that even though your body is upright, your posture should remain alive and not rigid.

Shoulders: The head should be pressed upward. The shoulders should be dropped downward. (When) the left shoulder turns, the right shoulder should follow automatically. When the body's Li is reaching to the hands, it is caused by the shoulders.

肩：頭宜上頂，肩宜下垂。左肩成拗，右肩自隨。身力
到手，肩之所為。

This second song talks about the postures of the head and the shoulders. When the head is pressed upward, it will feel suspended and the spirit of vitality can be raised. The shoulders should be dropped naturally and not tensed. The two shoulders should coordinate with each other closely. When one is moving, the other should naturally follow. In this case, the movement of the upper body can be smooth and the shoulders will be able to direct the Jin to the hands efficiently.

Arms: (When) the left am is extended, the right arm should be under the armpit. Like curved but not curved, like straight but not straight. Bend too much (and you) cannot reach far, and overly straight has less power.

臂：左臂前伸，右臂在肋。似曲不曲，似直不直。過曲
不遠，過直少力。

This song talks about the posture of the arms. When one arm is extended for striking or for intercepting, the other should take the responsibility of protecting the body. The key to doing this is dropping the elbow. The elbow can then protect the armpit, and the hand and forearm can easily protect the chest area. You should not bend your arm too much when you attack or protect yourself. When you bend too much, you will not be able to reach far for your attack, and when you block you will allow your opponent's attack too close to your body. However, if you keep your arm too straight, then the Jin cannot be stored efficiently. Also, if you extend your arm too far when you attack, the technique will lose some of its power.

Hands: The right hand is at the side under the armpit and the left hand is as high as the chest. The rear (arm) is bent slightly and the front (arm) extends strongly. Two hands cover all, and the use of Li should be appropriate.

手：右手在脅，左手齊胸。後者微塌，前者力伸。兩手
皆覆，用力宜勻。

This song describes the position of the arms in the basic ready posture. The body is turned somewhat to the right to give the opponent a smaller target, the right hand is held defensively below the left armpit, and the right arm is held extended with the hand at chest height. The right arm should be slightly bent so that it is ready to move in any direction, and the Yi of your left arm should extend strongly out to the front so that your spirit is high and your Qi is mobilized and ready. Your two hands cover the entire space in front of you, ready to attack or defend as necessary, and you should only use as much force (Li) as is necessary.

Fingers: Five fingers are separated and they are shaped like hooks. The tiger's mouth is round and full. (They are) like stiff like soft, the Li must be able to reach the fingers and must not be forced.

指：五指各分，其形似鉤。虎口圓滿，似剛似柔。力須
到指，不可強求。

When your hands are open, the fingers should be separated, but not too far apart. The fingers should be bent like hooks, and the tiger mouth area (between the thumb and index finger)(Hu Kou, 虎口) should be round and full of Qi. Though the hand looks powerful, it is not tensed, because that would prevent the Qi from reaching the fingertips and would hinder the manifesting of Li.

Thighs: The left thigh is in front and the right thigh is supporting in the rear. Like straight but not straight, like bowed but not bowed, although there is straight and bent, every (move you) always see the chicken shape.

股：左股在前，右股後撐。似直不直，似弓不弓。雖有
直曲，每見雞形。

In Xingyiquan you will normally have most of your weight on your rear leg. Both legs should be slightly bent. This posture is considered the chicken shape in Xingyiquan.

Feet: Left foot straight forward, leaning sideways is all sick. The posture of the right foot is at an angle. The front heel faces the (rear) shin. The distance (between the feet) is according to the individual. The toes are arcing inward to firm (the root).

足：左足直前，斜側皆病。右足勢斜，前踵對脛。隨人
距離，足趾扣定。

When your left foot is forward, it should point in the direction your body is facing, i.e., slightly to the right. This turns your knee in slightly to protect your groin. Your rear foot should be at an angle, pointing to your fight front. The stance is narrow, with the heel of the front foot in front of the rear leg (shin).

> *Tongue: The tongue is the extremity of the meat (i.e., muscle). (When it is) curved, then the Qi is sunk. The eyes wide open and the hair sticking up. (When the Qi) is sunk more to the (Lower) Dan Tian, the facial skin is like iron and the viscera and bowels are solid internally.*

> 舌：舌為肉梢，捲則氣降。目張髮聳，丹田愈沉。肌容如鐵，內堅五臟。

When the tongue is curved upward to touch the roof of the mouth, the Qi can be sunk. This will also raise up the spirit of vitality so that the eyes are wide open and the Qi can reach the hair and make it stand on end. If the Qi can be sunk more fully to the Lower Dan Tian, the Qi can reach the skin more efficiently and make the skin as strong as iron, and the internal organs strong and solid.

> *Hips: (When) the hips are raised, the Qi will reach the four extremities. The two legs are twisting around and the meat contacts on the buttocks. (If) the posture is too low, then the shape is loose, therefore, it should be slightly higher.*

> 臀：提起臀部，氣貫四梢。兩眼繚繞，臀部肉交。低則勢散，故宜稍高。

When the buttocks are slightly tensed ("raised") and the two sides pressed together, the Qi can be raised to reach the four extremities: the tongue, hair, nails, and teeth. In Qigong practice, the Huiyin (會陰) cavity and the anus are held up in order to lead the Qi upward to reach the head and the limbs. When you are holding up the Huiyin and anus, the buttocks will also be raised and slightly tensed, and the two sides will be pressed together. The legs are twisted slightly inward in order to firm your root and stabilize your stance. In addition, your stance should not be too high or too low. The best stance is the one in which you feel most comfortable and can manifest your Jin most strongly.

2.3 SUMMARY OF KEY POINTS

It does not matter which internal Chinese martial art you learn, the basic training theory and principles remain the same. The different styles are simply different ways of approaching the final goal. Before we discuss the key points of Xingyiquan, it would be a good idea to first review the general theory and principles which these internal arts have in common. For a more detailed discussion of these, please refer to the book, *Tai Chi Theory and Martial Power,* by Dr. Yang.

2.3.1 General Theory of the Internal Styles

A. **Training the Qi body is more important than training the physical body.** Learning how to build up the Qi, circulate it, and apply it to the physical body is the major concern in almost all of the internal martial arts styles. Only after the Qi has been built to a higher level can it be used to energize the physical body and be coordinated with the techniques to make them more efficient and effective.

B. **Yin and Yang balance.** In order to build up the Qi body harmoniously, you must be concerned with balancing Yin and Yang. If you neglect this and train improperly, your body can become excessively Yin or Yang, and you can cause yourself physical or mental injury. Yin and Yang theory is also commonly used to analyze strategy, techniques, and the manifestation of Jin. For example, storage is Yin and manifestation is Yang. Yin and Yang theory is one of the most basic roots of the internal arts.

C. **Yin and Yang combine.** Once you understand the theory of balancing Yin and Yang, then you must also learn how to bring them together and make them interact. The combining of Yin and Yang creates all things and all variations. In the Qi body the main concern is how to use Kan (坎) (Water) and Li (離)(Fire) to adjust the body's Yin and Yang, and how to cause them to interact in a harmonious and balanced fashion. In strategy, techniques, and the manifestation of Jin, when Yin and Yang are combined the strategy can be alive and your intentions can be hidden from the opponent, the techniques can be varied from substantial to insubstantial or vice versa easily, and finally the Jin can have a firm, balanced root so that it is strong. You can see that you need to balance Yin and Yang to keep everything neutral, and you need to combine Yin and Yang to demonstrate their power. It is like the positive and negative charges in electricity: when you bring them together you can manifest power and run machines.

D. **The manifestation of Jin.** Because Xingyiquan is a martial art, manifesting maximum power is of major concern right from the beginning of the training. The manifestation of Jin can be analyzed according to Yin and Yang theory. For example, Yin is storing the Jin (in the Yi, Qi, and posture) and Yang is manifesting the Jin. When you store your Jin, you must first store it in your Yi (the level-headed, judging part of your mind). This makes it possible to store the Qi and condense it in the Lower Dan Tian and bone marrow. Storing the Yi and Qi are internal and cannot be seen. Storing Jin is like drawing a bow before you shoot. The more efficiently you can store Jin in your Yi, Qi, and posture, the more strongly you will be able to manifest the power. In order to manifest what you have stored externally, your physical body must utilize a posture which can most strongly express the Jin. When the Jin is manifested, you must again be concerned with how to balance it. For example, when you push a car, you must also push backward in order to have any forward power. Therefore, when Jin is manifested, Yin and Yang are again involved.

E. **General concepts in training.** Qigong (氣功)(i.e., the study of Qi) is one of the most important areas trained in every Chinese internal martial style. Generally, there are five steps in reaching the final goal of spiritual cultivation in the martial arts: 1. regulating the body; 2. regulating the breathing; 3. regulating the mind (Yi and Xin); 4. regulating the Chi; and 5. regulating the spirit. In fact, these five steps are common to all Chinese Qigong training. For a more detailed discussion please refer to the book, *The Root of Chinese Qigong*, by Dr. Yang.

2.3.2 The Root and Essence of Xingyiquan Theory

A. **Qi is threaded through the entire body.** Like most other internal styles, Xingyiquan emphasizes using the "one Qi" to thread through the entire body. This means that the Qi unifies the body from top to bottom, both internally and externally.

B. **Yin and Yang combine.** Like other internal martial arts, Xingyiquan emphasizes the combination of Yin and Yang so that they coordinate and interact with each other harmoniously. Naturally, this must be built on a condition of balanced Yin and Yang.

C. **External and Internal combine.** The external means the physical manifestation (shape) and the internal means the thinking (mind), the Qi body, and the spirit. Internal (Yin) feeling and storage (storage of Yi, Qi, and spirit) are the foundation of the manifestation of the physical body (Yang). When these two are unified naturally, the entire body (both physical body and Qi body) can act and react as one unit.

D. **Six Unifications.** In order to reach the goal of mutual coordination, the six unifications are emphasized. These six unifications are divided into three external and three internal unifications. The three external unifications are the hands and the feet unify, the elbows and the knees unify, and the shoulder and the hips unify. The feet are the foundation which enables the Jin to be manifested strongly through the hands. Similarly, the knees and the hips are the foundations of the elbows and shoulders. The feet, knees, and hips are Yin and support the hands, elbows, and shoulders, which are the Yang. When the Qi originates in the Lower Dan Tian, one flow moves upward to the arms and the other flow downward to the legs. These two flows must balance each other in order for the Jin to manifest most strongly You can see that the three external unifications do not refer only to a physical coordination. The Qi must be expanded through the same areas and be coordinated or unified with them.

The three internal unifications refer to the unification of the Xin and Yi (emotional mind and wisdom mind), the Yi and Qi, and finally Qi and Li. In a fight, you must have a clear mind and wise judgement before you can use your mind to lead the Qi efficiently (Yi and Qi unify) to energize the muscles to maximum power (Qi and Li unify). The first step is the wisdom mind learning how to control the emotional mind so that the two minds act as one.

E. **Theory of the Five Phases.** The most unique part of Xingyiquan theory is the application of the Five Phases. The five basic strategic movements were created out of the relationships of mutual production and conquest of the Five Phases. These five basic movements are not only the foundation of the fighting techniques and strategy, but they are also an effective way of regulating the Qi in the five viscera.

2.3.3 Regulating the Body in Xingyiquan

A. **Basic requirements.** 1. The body is centered and balanced; 2. the head is pressed upward to raise up the spirit of vitality; 3. the shoulders are dropped, and both sides are coordinated; 4. the arms are slightly bent and the elbows are dropped; 5. the hands are in a line and coordinated with the knees; 6. the fingers are shaped like hooks, the tiger mouth area and the backs of the hands are rounded; 7. the two hips support each other and the thighs are shaped like a pair of scissors (chicken shape); 8. the feet are not far apart, the front toes are turned slightly inward and the bottoms of the feet grab the ground to firm the root; 9. the tongue is curved upward to connect the Yin and Yang Qi vessels.

B. **The basic stationary posture and the five basic movements.** The basic stationary posture is the three body posture (San Ti Shi, 三體式). Through this posture the mind is calm, the Qi is full, and the strength of the foundation is built. The five basic movements are Pi, Zuan, Beng, Pao, and Heng, and they are related to each other through the theory of the Five Phases.

C. **The key words are:** Ding (頂)(press), Ti (提)(hold up), Kou (扣)(arc/grab), Yuan (圓)(round), Bao (抱)(embrace), Chui (垂)(drop), Heng (橫)(sideways), Shun (順)(smoothness), Zuan (鑽)(drill), Fan (翻)(turn over), Min (敏)(acute), Qu (曲)(bend), and Ting (挺)(thrust).

2.3.4 Regulating the Breathing in Xingyiquan

Except for Yue, Fei's second thesis (Appendix A), there is almost nothing about breathing in the available documents. Since Xingyiquan is an internal Qigong style, the breathing, which is considered the strategy of Qigong training, should not be ignored. Normally speaking, there are two common ways of breathing trained in Qigong practice. One is normal deep abdominal breathing and the other is reverse deep abdominal breathing.

Normal abdominal breathing can make the muscles which control the expanding and contracting of the lungs more relaxed. This allows the lungs to expand more and take in more oxygen. This type of breathing also enables you to lead your mind into a more calm and relaxed meditative state.

However, when you intend to lead the Qi to the limbs to energize the muscles and manifest their power, then you must use the reverse abdominal breathing. Many people think that reverse abdominal breathing is against the way of "Dao" (道) (nature), but this is not true. If you experiment with pushing a heavy object with one hand while holding the other hand on your abdomen, you will see that as you push hard your abdomen will automatically expand. This is reverse breathing. It was discovered that in order to store Qi deep in the marrow, and also to manifest Jin most efficiently in the limbs, the best way is to use reverse breathing in coordination with inhaling and exhaling to lead the Qi inward and outward. This is why Yue, Fei's second thesis says that the inhale is Yin (storage) and the exhale is Yang (manifestation).

You should also understand that in order to condense Qi into the marrow and expand it out to the limbs and the surface of the skin efficiently, anus coordination is necessary. This is necessary to both build up Yin and Yang and to coordinate them. Since there is not too much information in the available documents, you should refer to other sources, such as Taijiquan, to obtain more knowledge of breathing.

2.3.5 Regulating the Mind in Xingyiquan

Before moving, the mind is in the Wuji (無極) state. In this state the mind is calm, neutral, and centered. On starting to move, the mind (or thoughts) are distinguished into Yin and Yang. Normally, the emotional mind (Xin, 心) is generated first from your feelings, and it is then regulated and judged by the wisdom mind (Yi, 意). Then you start to act.

One very significant difference between Xingyiquan and other internal martial Qigong or general Qigong is in the regulating of the mind. Generally in Qigong it is desirable that the emotional mind be completely suppressed and dominated by the wisdom mind (Yi). This means that emotional feelings are limited to a minimum while the mind is being regulated and cultivated. However, in Xingyiquan the emotional mind should not be suppressed. On the contrary, it is encouraged and stimulated to a higher state of excitement. For example, it says that the mind is like a fiery tiger which is able to excite your feelings and raise up your spirit so that you will not be afraid. The reason for doing this goes back to the fact that Xingyiquan imitates animals. Because animals don't have a high level of wisdom mind, when they fight they react naturally, from their feelings. In order to unite your mind and your techniques, you cannot suppress the emotional mind.

However, although the emotional mind is allowed to develop to a high level in Xingyiquan, the wisdom mind (Yi) must still be cultivated until it is able to control the emotional mind and coordinate with it. The emotional mind is like a wild and fierce tiger, and the wisdom mind is the animal tamer. You would like to control and govern it so that it can act properly in a fight, but you do not want to completely tame the tiger so that it loses its wild, original nature.

You can see that the hardest part of the training in Xingyiquan is probably the regulating of the mind. The emotional mind is Yang and the wisdom mind is Yin, and although they are the opposite of each other, and often oppose each other, they must be coordinated and balanced with each other to work together harmoniously.

2.3.6 Regulating the Qi in Xingyiquan

Regardless of which style of Qigong you are training, you are learning how to convert Essence into Qi (Lian Jing Hua Qi, 練精化氣), to lead the Qi upward to the head to nourish the brain and spirit (Lian Qi Hua Shen, 練氣化神), and finally to train the spirit to be independent and enter the world of no desire (nothingness)(Lian Shen Huan Xu, 練神返虛). It is the same for Xingyiquan. The first step is learning how to regulate the body, breathing, mind, and then Qi, the second step is learning how to raise up your spirit to a higher state, and finally the last step is aiming for enlightenment or Buddhahood. Naturally, in Xingyiquan Qigong, you must follow the same procedures and aim for the final goal of calmness and peacefulness.

Most beginners, in order to reach the final goal of the cultivation, must first learn the unification of the external physical body and the internal viscera. You should understand that the primary Qi channels connect the viscera to the limbs. From the point of view of Qi, they are closely related and cannot be separated. One part of Xingyiquan training is to thread the Qi through the entire body and make the body feel and act as one. In order to reach this goal, the physical body and the internal mind, feeling, and spirit must be united. Only then can the Qi move freely and smoothly without stagnation. Once you have reached a higher level where you concentrate on the Qi body, the physical body will gradually seem to disappear and become transparent.

The next step in Xingyiquan is to lead an abundant amount of Qi to the four extremities (tongue, hair, nails, and teeth). If you can do this efficiently you have proven that the Qi in your body is abundant and can be directed by your Yi as desired.

Finally, Xingyiquan also emphasizes the regulation of Qi in the five most vital Yin viscera or organs (heart, lungs, liver, kidneys, and spleen). Regulating the Qi smoothly and to an accurate level in the five organs is one of the main goals in Qigong practice. This process of leading the Qi in the five organs to the proper or "original" level is called "Wu Qi Chao Yuan" (五氣朝元)(The five Qi's are led toward their origins). In Xingyiquan, the five basic movements are designed (along with the help of your Xin and Yi) to smooth out the Qi in these five organs. For example, in the Pao movement, you imitate a cannon firing. The movement is fast and straight forward, with one arm rising as the other punches directly ahead. This movement rapidly contracts and expands the area of the heart and lungs, increasing the Qi circulation there. Furthermore, your Xin and Yi are involved in imagining the feeling of a cannon firing, which enables you to lead the Qi more efficiently.

2.3.7 Regulating the Spirit in Xingyiquan

When you are in a fight, your spirit is alert and sharp like an eagle's. When you are calm, your mind is calm and peaceful. The final goal is to reach enlightenment. One of the documents points out the procedures for approaching this goal. It says: "(When) the Xin (emotional mind) is steady, the Shen (spirit) is calm. The Shen is calm, the Xin is peaceful. The Xin is peaceful, then it is quiet and clean. It is quiet and clean, then nothing exists. When nothing exists, the Qi will be transported (smoothly). When Qi is transported smoothly, then the imagination disappears. When the imagination disappears, then the feeling (i.e., sensing) is clear. When the feeling is clear, then the Shen and Qi are mutually connected. In this case, millions of Qis return to their roots."

2.3.8 The Strategy of Xingyiquan

Xingyiquan adopts the relationship of mutual production and conquest in the Five Phases to form the five basic movements. Out of this relationship are developed the various techniques. The manner of fighting and the techniques of the twelve animals were combined with these five basic movements into a very effective style.

Xingyiquan emphasizes advancing and withdrawing in a straight line, although sideward movements and dodging are also used to prepare for the advance. Xingyiquan uses offense as the defense. Aggressive attacking and advancing are the main objectives of the training.

2.3.9 The Key Trainings of Xingyiquan

In order to make the strategy and techniques effective, seven "speeds" are emphasized in the training. These are: the eyes are speedy, the hands are speedy, the feet are speedy, the Yi is speedy, the attack is speedy, advancing and withdrawing are speedy, the body's movements are speedy.

In order to make all of the strategic movements and techniques become natural reactions, you must train until you have accomplished the goal of the seven smooth movements of the physical body These seven smoothnesses are: 1. The shoulders should urge (i.e., push) the elbows, and the elbows should not oppose the shoulders; 2. The elbows should urge the hands, and the hands should not oppose the elbows; 3. The hands should urge the fingers, and the fingers should not oppose the hands; 4. The waist should urge the hips, and the hips should not oppose the waist; 5. The hips should urge the knees, and the knees should not oppose the hips; 6. The knees should urge the feet, and the feet should not oppose the knees; 7. The head should urge the body, and the body should not oppose the head.

The documents also mention the eight importances of Xingyiquan. These are: inside must be lifted, the three centers must be together, the three Yis must be linked together, the Five Phases must be smooth, the four extremities must be uniform, the Xin must be leisurely, the three tips must face each other, and finally the eyes must be venomous.

2.3.10 The Jins of Xingyiquan

Xingyiquan uses many different patterns of Jin, but five of them are particularly emphasized. These five are: Cai (踩)(stepping), Pu (撲)(leap), Guo (裹)(enwrapping), Shu (束)(binding)(i.e., sealing), and Jue (決)(thrusting). It is said: "Cai Jin (Stepping Jin) is like stepping on something poisonous. Pu Jin (Leaping Jin) is like the leaping of the rabbit and the tiger. Guo Jin (Enwrapping Jin) is like wrapping something so that nothing is exposed. Shu Jin (Binding Jin) is like binding the top and the bottom into one. Jue Jin (Thrusting Jin) is like water breaking through a dam. The Stepping needs the Thrusting, the Leaping needs the Thrusting, the Enwrapping needs the Thrusting, The Thrusting needs the Thrusting. One Thrusting, not one without thrust. If there is no thrusting, there is no agility"

References

1. "形意拳圖說" (*The Illustration of Xingyiquan*), Ling, Gui-Qing (凌桂青), Reprinted in Taipei, Taiwan, 1929.

2. "形意母拳" (*The Mother Fist of Xingyiquan*), Jiang, Rong-Qiao (姜容樵), Reprinted in Taipei, Taiwan, 1929.

CHAPTER 3

Xingyi Qigong 形意氣功

3.1 ABOUT XINGYI QIGONG

Since Da Mo (達磨) wrote his two Qigong classics at the Shaolin Temple around 550 A.D., experience has shown that Qigong can not only improve the health of a martial artist, it can also significantly increase the power and enhance the effectiveness of his martial techniques. Qigong has become a necessary part of the training in every style of Chinese martial arts.

Naturally, Xingyiquan, as an internal style with its main emphasis on Qi development, has its own ways of training Qi. Since the creation of Xingyiquan, many masters have created Qigong sets for the art. Although the forms are different, the purpose and the basic training theory remain the same. In this chapter we will introduce the training sets created by Master Zhang, Zhao-Dong (張兆東).

Once you have mastered this set, you should not feel that you must restrict yourself to only these few forms. After practicing and studying for a long time, if you really comprehend Qigong theory and Xingyiquan, you may be able to modify the existing forms or even create new ones which are more effective in improving your health and increasing the effectiveness of your Xingyiquan. However, you must recognize that it is not easy to reach this high level of understanding.

The principles and training theory of all forms of Chinese Qigong are built on three roots: Jing (精)(Essence), Qi (氣)(internal bioelectric energy), and Shen (神 (spirit). For health purposes, the goal of your training is to learn how to maintain smooth Qi circulation in the twelve primary Qi channels (Shi Er Jing, 十二經) and how to fill the eight Qi vessels (八脈) with an abundant level of Qi. As a martial artist you also learn how to apply the Qi to the techniques to make them more powerful and effective. That means combining the internal energy and the external physical body into one.

Whether you train Qigong for health or for martial arts, you have to learn how to increase the efficiency with which you convert Jing (Essence) into Qi, and also learn how to lead Qi to your head to nourish your brain, which allows you to raise up your spirit of vitality. This, in turn, enables you to increase your power to its maximum.

Qigong training typically begins with learning how to regulate the body, followed by the breathing, emotional mind, Qi, and finally Shen. Since this is an

Figure 3-1

Figure 3-2

extensive and profound subject, it is impossible to discuss it in only a few pages of this book. If you are interested in Chinese Qigong, you should read: *The Root of Chinese Qigong,* by Dr. Yang.

3.2 Xingyi Qigong Training

In this section we will introduce twelve Xingyi Qigong exercises.

1. Pick Up the Moon from Sea Bottom (Hai Di Lao Yue, 海底撈月):

Movements: Standing in a Horse Stance (Ma Bu, 馬步), let your hands drop naturally to your sides (Figure 3-1). Inhale and exhale twenty times, and then shake your entire body like a dog off shaking water. Inhale, then exhale with a deep, loud cough. Turn your palms face down and then lower your body. Your hands press downward until they are only a couple of inches from the ground (Figure 3-2). Move your hands in circles beside your feet, first clockwise and then counterclockwise (Figure 3-3). Close your fists, imagine that you are holding a heavy object, and lift it up over your head while standing up (Figure 3-4). Your head tilts back to look upward as you do this. Next, inhale and bend your knees while your hands are still over your head and the head is looking upward (Figure 3-5). Exhale and then inhale while opening your hands and moving them to the sides with the palms facing upward (Figure 3-6). Extend your two arms to the sides and circle them to the sides of your

Figure 3-3

Figure 3-4

Figure 3-5

Figure 3-6

Figure 3-7   Figure 3-8

face (Figure 3-7), and press them down again to the beginning posture. Repeat twenty times.

Purpose: To build up the strength of the knees and strengthen the foundation of your stance. This exercise also trains you to lead Qi to your hands in coordination with the movements.

2. Lion Turns the Ball (Shi Zi Tuan Qiu, 獅子搏球):

Movements: Standing in a Horse Stance, inhale and fill up your Dan Tian with Qi. Both hands move up to the level of the navel, with the palms facing up (Figure 3-8). Your hands are curved as if you were holding a ball in each hand. Extend your right hand forward while exhaling and turning your body slightly (Figure 3-9), and then turn the right hand downward (Yin palm, 陰掌) while inhaling and moving it back to the waist area (Figure 3-10). Then extend and draw back your left hand the same way. As you are doing this, your body should turn naturally and smoothly in coordination with the movement of the hands. Repeat twenty times.

Purpose: To loosen up the waist area and learn how to use the Yi to lead the Qi to the extending hands. These movements will also strengthen the chest and shoulders.

Figure 3-9

Figure 3-10

Figure 3-11

Figure 3-12

3. Spiritual Dragon Turns His Head (Shen Long Hui Shou, 神龍回首 *):*

Movements: Stand in a Horse Stance with the two hands dropped naturally at your sides (Figure 3-11). Raise your right hand, palm upward as if you were holding something, and simultaneously raise your left hand, but with the palm facing downward. When they reach the height of your stomach, the palms turn toward each other (Figure 3-12). Without stopping the motion, turn your body to the left while the right hand continues to move upward diagonally leftward, while the left hand presses diagonally downward to the rear (Figure 3-13). Finally, turn your body back to the front with your left hand on the bottom palm up and the fight hand on the top palm facing down (Figure 3-14). Turn your body to the right and reverse the motions. Repeat twenty times.

Purpose: The twisting movement loosens up the trunk, while the holding up and pressing down of the hands trains the Qi to expand diagonally.

Figure 3-13

Figure 3-14

4. Open and Close to Rotate the Eyeballs (Kai He Lun Jing, 開合輪睛):

Movements: Stand upright with the feet slightly apart and the hands dropped naturally, and relax completely. The head is pressing upward (i.e., the head is suspended). With the eyes closed, rotate your eyeballs clockwise twenty times and then counterclockwise twenty times. Then repeat the same rotations with your eyes open (Figure 3-15).

Purpose: To exercise the muscles controlling the eyeballs. This increases the circulation of Qi around the eyes and slows the deterioration of the eyes.

Figure 3-15

Figure 3-16

Figure 3-17

5. Look to the Left and Beware of the Right (Zuo Gu Yao Pan, 左顧右盼 *):*

Movements: Continuing from the last form, first inhale, and then turn your head to the left to the maximum while exhaling (Figure 3-16), then turn your head to the front while inhaling. Repeat the same movement to the right. While you are inhaling, store Qi in the Lower Dan Tian, and while you are exhaling, lead the Qi to the skin, to the limbs, and to the head. Repeat twenty times.

Purpose: To loosen and stretch the neck muscles, and loosen up the Qi channels which pass through the neck.

6. Large Python Swings Its Head (Da Mang Yao Tou, 大蟒搖頭 :

Movements: Continuing from the last form, interlock your hands and place them behind your head. Use your arms to move the head to the right in a circular motion twenty times (Figure 3-17), and then repeat the same movements to the left. Do not circle on too large of a scale. If you do, the vertebra in the lower section of the neck will be pressed and ground away causing damage or arthritis.

Purpose: To loosen up the neck and increase the Qi and blood circulation in the neck and shoulders.

Figure 3-18

Figure 3-19

7. Rinse the Ears and Eyes (Er Mu Shuang Di, 耳目雙滌):

Movements: Continuing from the last movement, rub your hands until they are very warm. Use both hands to rub the forehead (Figure 3-18), both temples (Figure 3-19), and the top of your head (Figure 3-20). Rub the inner sides of the eyes with your middle fingers (Figure 3-21), and then rub the area around your ears with your index fingers (Figure 3-22). Repeat the entire procedure three times.

Purpose: To use the Qi generated from rubbing the hands to nourish the head and smooth out the Qi. The rubbing increases the Qi and blood circulation around the eyes and ears, and keeps them functioning in a healthy manner.

Figure 3-20

Figure 3-21

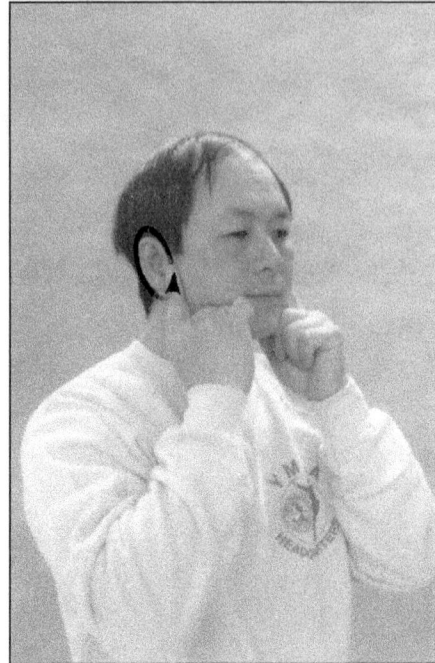

Figure 3-22

8. Listen to the Organ Three Times (San Du Ting Guan, 三度聽官):

Movements: Continuing from the last form, rub your hands again until they are very warm, and cover your ears tightly (Figure 3-23). Pause for a few seconds, then suddenly remove the hands from the ears (Figure 3-24). Repeat twice more.

Purpose: To maintain your hearing.

Figure 3-23

Figure 3-24

9. Rub the Tendons Behind the Brain (Nao Hou Zhai Jin, 腦後摘筋):

Movements: Continuing from the last form, again rub your hands until they are very warm. Then drop your left hand naturally and use your fight hand to rub and slide down the back of your head and neck (Figure 3-25) three times. Rub your hands again and repeat but with the hands reversed.

Purpose: To increase the Qi and blood circulation from the neck to the brain.

Figure 3-25

Figure 3-26

Figure 3-27

10. Beat the Drum Nine Times (Er Gu Jiu Za, 耳鼓九匝):

Movements: Continuing from the last form, use the fingers of your right hand to brush your right ear three times (Figure 3-26), then press on the hole in the ear with your middle finger three times (Figure 3-27), and finally use your palm to push the ear down to cover the hole in the ear, and lightly snap your index finger off the middle finger to tap on your head several times (Figure 3-28). Repeat the same procedure on your left side.

Purpose: To maintain proper functioning and to increase the Qi and blood circulation in your ears.

Figure 3-28

Figure 3-29

11. Hen and Ha Two Qis (Hen Ha Er Qi, 哼哈二氣):

Movements: Continuing from the last form, stare at your thumbs and concentrate on them as you rub them together until they are warm (Figure 3-29). Then raise your head to face upward and rub the sides of the lower part of your nose with your thumbs (Figure 3-30). Repeat the entire process one more time.

Purpose: To increase the Qi and blood circulation in the sinus area.

Figure 3-30

*12. Exhale the Dew to Thread the Sun
(Xu Lu Guan Ri, 嘘露貫日):*

Movements: Continuing from the last form, rub your hands until they are very warm, then rub your head, face, and temples. Then brush your hands, one at a time, down the front of your body to your Lower Dan Tian several times as if you were brushing a long beard. As you are doing this, look upward, inhale deeply and then exhale (Figure 3-31).

Purpose: After circulating the Qi in the face area, lead it down to the Lower Dan Tian.

Figure 3-31

CHAPTER 4
Fundamental Moving Patterns 基本五拳

4.1 INTRODUCTION

We will begin this chapter by introducing the most basic stationary posture of Xingyiquan, the three body posture (San Ti Shi, 三體式). This posture is also commonly called the three power posture (San Cai Shi, 三才式) or Taiji posture (Taiji Shi, 太極式). The main purpose of this stationary stance is to build up your physical strength and to train beginners in correct standing posture. It helps the beginner to understand the basic requirements of Xingyiquan, such as the three external unifications and the three internal unifications. This posture is also used for bringing the mind into a peaceful, calm, and natural state. Only when you feel natural and comfortable in this stance will you be able to move smoothly and naturally.

After you feel comfortable in the three body posture, you should then learn the five basic movements. Since they correspond to the Five Phases (Wu Xing, 五行), they are therefore called "Wu Xing" or "five phases movements." They are also commonly called "Wu Quan" (五拳), which means "the five fists." These five fists are Pi Quan (劈拳), Zuan Quan (鑽拳), Beng Quan (弸拳), Pao Quan (炮拳), and Heng Quan (橫拳). Each fist is related to the Qi circulation in one of the five viscera. Qi is Yin in comparison to the physical body, which is Yang. When Yin is smooth, the Yang will be strong and healthy. Yin is the foundation of Yang, and Yang is the manifestation of Yin. Training these five basic movements teaches the beginner how to unify the internal Qi and the external physical movements.

Before we introduce these movements, you should first learn these important points and precautions:

1. The best time to practice Xingyiquan is at dawn when the environmental and bodily Qi is changing from Yin to Yang.

2. One hour of practice each time is adequate. Longer than one hour and you will lose your concentration and the feeling for the exercises. In addition, you will become tired and will start to lose the coordination between your body and mind.

3. Do not practice right after a meal. Instead, wait a few hours.

4. Do not practice when you are hungry.

5. Practice five minutes and rest for five minutes until the body and the mind return to their original state. When you rest, do not sit down. Simply walk around slowly.

6. Right after practice, do not expose your body to the wind. You may catch cold.

7. The air should be fresh and circulating in the practice area.

8. Do not practice right after drinking alcohol. Do not smoke or eat during the practice session.

9. Do not practice when you are upset, because your mind will be disturbed and Qi circulation will not be smooth.

4.2 THE THREE BODY POSTURE

The Three Body Posture (San Ti Shi) 三體式

1. Stand straight with your arms dropped naturally to your sides, look forward, and keep your mind in the Wuji state. Your tongue should touch the roof of your mouth (Figure 4-1).

2. Keep the left foot in place and turn your whole body and right foot 45 degrees to the right (Figure 4-2).

3. Raise both arms to the level of your chest, with the right hand on top of the left hand, and bend your knees slightly. The right index finger is lined up with the left middle finger (Figure 4-3).

4. Push your left hand upward and forward as you bring the right hand down to your abdomen, bending your wrists so that the fingers point up, and at the same time step forward with your left leg (Figure 4-4). The fingers are open, the back of the hands are round, and the tiger mouths (Hu Kou, 虎口) (space between thumb and index finger) are also round. The hands, the front foot, and the nose should line up. The eyes are concentrating and staring forward, and the Qi is sunk. Your weight is 60% on the rear leg. Having one hand touch your abdomen in front of the Dan Tian helps you to focus and accumulate your Qi there.

You should train standing in this posture for at least ten minutes to half an hour each time. This is necessary to build up the strength of your legs and arms so that the posture can be natural and comfortable, and also to train your mind to be calm and peaceful and unified with the posture. During the course of practicing Xingyiquan you should frequently go back to Chapter 2 and read the documents which have been passed down through generations. They explain the criteria and the theoretical foundation of your practice.

Figure 4-1

Figure 4-2

Figure 4-3

Figure 4-4

4.3 Pi Quan

Pi (劈) in Chinese has the meaning of splitting, rending, or cleaving. However, none of these words expresses the actual meaning (action and feeling) completely. Some of these words lack the feeling of the actual action (attacking), while others miss the feeling of tearing apart. When doing Pi, the front hand is formed like an ax and chops down on something. However, in the actual movement, the chopping force is not exactly downward; instead, it is forward and downward. While the front hand is making this motion, the rear hand is drawing in to the abdomen. This gives the feeling of using both hands to rend or tear something apart.

When you make the Pi movement, and, in fact, when you do any of the five movements, one hand pulls in to the abdomen. This balances the physical movement of the other arm, but it also helps you to draw Qi into your Lower Dan Tian and accumulate it there. Since it causes you to continually pay attention to your Lower Dan Tian, it also helps you to make all of your movements start from it, and draw their energy from it.

As mentioned in the second chapter, Pi and each of the other four fists are different patterns of movement for expressing Jin (勁), instead of a specific action. Pi can be any one of several movements, but it must always have its characteristic pattern or feeling through which the Jin is manifested.

The available documents have two sections and two songs which explain the Pi pattern.

About Pi Quan #1 劈拳說一

Pi Quan belongs to Metal and is the raising and falling of "One Qi." Pi, because the movement of its hand is like an ax chopping, therefore belongs to Metal in the theory of the Five Phases. Its shape is like an ax, and belongs to the lungs in the body and (manifests) in the fist as Pi (chopping). (When) its Jin is smooth, the lungs' Qi will be harmonious, and (if) the Jin is incorrect, then the lungs' Qi will be weird. A man('s life) is mastered with Qi, and when Qi is harmonious, then the body is strong, and when Qi is weird, then the body is weak. Therefore, Pi Quan is used as the first (training) in Xingyiquan, it is considering that Yang Qi (nourishing Qi) is the most important.

> 劈拳屬金，是一氣之起落也。劈者，以其掌之下，如斧
> 之劈也。故於五行之理屬金。其形像斧，在腹內則屬肺，
> 在拳即為劈。其勁順，則肺氣和，其勁謬，則肺氣乖。
> 人以氣為主，氣和則體壯，氣乖則體弱。故形意拳以劈
> 拳為首，即以養氣為先務也。

Pi Quan corresponds to the lungs in the Five Phases and therefore belongs to Metal. When Metal is cold, it is able to cool down the Fire Qi, and when it is hot, it is able to raise up the Qi. When you perform Pi Quan, your hand is like an ax which is chopping down on something. From the Qigong point of view, the movement of Pi Quan is able to expand and compress the lungs. Therefore, when Pi Quan is performed smoothly both internally (i.e., Qi) and externally (movements), the lung Qi will be smooth. In this case, you will be able to absorb the oxygen (air essence) and convert it into Qi to nourish your body.

About Pi Quan #2 劈拳說二

The shape of Pi Quan is like an ax and belongs to Metal in the Five Phases. Therefore it is the leader of the Five Phases. When it is applied to the theory of mutual production, Pi Quan is able to produce Zuan Quan, (because) Metal is able to produce Water. When it is applied in the theory of mutual conquest, Pi Quan is able to conquer Beng Quan, (because) Metal is able to conquer Wood. If we discuss how it is hidden in the Five Phases, the lungs belong to Metal and when it is manifested externally, the nose is connected to the lungs. This is the theory of mutual production and conquest in the Five Phases, and it is also the theory of Pi Quan. Therefore, in Xingyiquan, Pi Quan is used as the first for those who begin to learn.

> 劈拳之形似斧，五行屬金。故為形意母拳之首。以相生
> 之理論之，劈拳能生鑽拳，金生水也。由相克之理論之，
> 劈拳能克弸拳，金克木也。以五行隱於內者言，肺屬金。
> 以五行著於外者言，鼻能通肺。此五行生克之理，劈拳
> 學之說也。故形意拳，以劈拳為五行之首，開始初學之
> 一，蓋基此也。

Metal is the first of the Five Phases (Figure 4-5). Therefore, Pi Quan is also considered the most basic and most important of the Five Fists. As a Xingyiquan beginner, you should first practice how to regulate your lungs. Only when the lungs can inhale and exhale smoothly and the lung Qi can circulate smoothly can the other four Jins be effectively manifested. Correct breathing is one of the most important keys in Qigong training.

Pi Quan Song #1 劈拳歌一

The two fists are like embracing and move toward the mouth. The fist is drilling upward the same height as the eyebrows. The latter fist (i.e., other hand) follows closely and connects tightly. The two arms are embracing the sides as high as the heart.

> 兩拳似抱口中去，拳前上鑽如眉齊。
> 後拳隨跟緊相連，兩手抱脅如心齊。

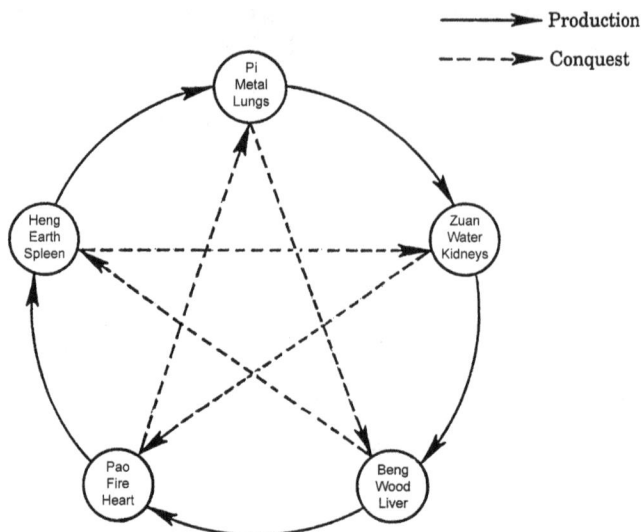

Figure 4-5. The relationships between the Five Phases

This section of the song describes the movements of Pi Quan. Raise your hands as if you were embracing something and continue upward toward the mouth. The first fist drills out from the center, rising to the height of the eyebrows. The other hand follows close behind, as if the hands were closely connected. At the completion of Pi Quan, the elbows are sunken to protect the sides and the front hand is as high as the heart.

The Qi falls to the Dan Tian following the body movements. Two hands fall together and the rear foot follows. Four fingers are open and the tiger mouth is round. The high and low of the front hand is the same as the heart.

氣隨身法落丹田，兩手齊落後腳隨。
四指分開虎口圓，前手高低與心齊。

Qi must be sunk to the Dan Tian, where it is accumulated during the storing part of the Jin movements. When the Jin of Pi Quan is manifested, both hands fall at the same time, and the rear leg follows the front leg as it steps forward. The fingers of both hands are opened and the space between the thumb and the second finger (tiger mouth)(Hu Kou, 虎口) is round. The front hand is as high as the heart and the rear hand is hidden below the armpit of the front hand.

The rear hand is always hidden under the armpit. The tips of the hands, (front) foot, and the nose are lined up. The little finger is turned upward as high as the eyebrows. The method of the Pi Quan strike is drilling upward. The feet and the hands fall together and the tongue is pressing upward. Step and exchange the forms, the Yin palm is falling.

後手只在脅下藏，手足鼻尖三對尖。
小指翻上如眉齊，劈拳打法向上鑽。
腳手齊落舌尖頂，進步換式陰掌落。

The tips of the hands, front foot, and nose should all be in the same plane. Some Xingyiquan masters believe that both feet should line up with the hands and nose. In this case, the tip of the front foot and the heel of the rear foot should line up. The fingers point upward. In the beginning of Pi Quan one hand drills up and forward, then the second hand chops forward and down for the strike. When striking, the hands and feet should fall together. The tongue should always touch the roof of the mouth. When you step forward to do the movement ("exchange the forms"), the palms face down and become Yin palms.

Pi Quan Song #2 劈拳歌二

Pi Quan is like an ax and its characteristics belong to Metal. (It) produces Zuan and conquers Beng, these (relations are) marvelous without peer. (When) the Metal is hidden internally, the nose is connected to the lungs. It is true that it is number one among the Five Phases.

劈拳似斧性屬金，生鑽克弸妙絕倫。
金隱於內鼻通肺，五行第一存其真。

This song repeats the relationship of Pi Quan to the Five Phases.

Figure 4-6

Figure 4-7

4.3.1 The Movements of Pi Quan:

Right Hand Pi:

1. Step into the three body posture (Figure 4-6).

2. Bring both hands to the abdomen, closing them into fists with the palms facing upward (Figure 4-7).

3. As you take a small step forward with your left foot, drill your left fist upward and forward to about face level (Figure 4-8).

4. As you step forward with your right leg, raise your right fist up to your chin and then thrust it out, turning and opening the palm so that the fingers point upward. At the same time bring the left hand down to the abdomen with the palm open and pulled back so that the fingers point up. The left foot then takes a small step to follow the right leg, and you shift 60% of your weight to it (Figure 4-9).

Left Hand Pi:

5. Bring both hands to the abdomen while closing the fists, palms facing upward (Figure 4-10).

6. The right hand moves from the abdomen up and out to the level of the face as you step forward with the right foot (Figure 4-11).

Figure 4-8

Figure 4-9

Figure 4-10

Figure 4-11

Figure 4-12

Figure 4-13

7. Move the left fist from the abdomen up to the chin and then out, opening the fist so that the fingers point up, while at the same time bringing the right hand down to the abdomen, with the palm open and fingers extended. As you do this, take a full step forward with your left leg, and let the right leg follow with a small step. Once the rear step follows, shift 60% of your weight to it (Figure 4-12).

Right Hand and Left Hand Pi can be repeated as many times as space allows. When you have run out of space, you may turn around and change your direction and continue your practice. The method of turning is very simple:

Changing Direction:

8. If you end with Left Hand Pi, pivot your left foot and shift all your weight to it, and turn clockwise. At the same time close your hands into fists and bring them to your waist, palms facing up (Figure 4-13). Then step your right leg forward and repeat the right hand Pi.

4.3.2 Application of Pi Quan:

In order to avoid confusion we will show only the beginning level applications. In the following explanations, you are the one with the black uniform using the Pi Quan. Start in the fighting posture with your left hand up and facing your opponent (Figure 4-14). When your opponent punches you with his right hand, intercept it with your right hand (Figure 4-15). Then grab his right wrist with your right hand and pull it down, while moving your left hand forward and downward to lock the opponent's shoulder (Figure 4-16). Alternatively, your left hand may attack diagonally upward to strike the opponent's neck (Figure 4-17) or press his shoulder joint down to dislocate the shoulder (Figure 4-18).

Figure 4-14

Figure 4-15

Figure 4-16

4.4 ZUAN QUAN

The Chinese word "Zuan" (鑽) means to drill, penetrate, and force one's way through. The motion is forward, aggressive, and it rotates like a drill. Though the motion is forward, it is usually also upward or downward. In Xingyiquan, the Zuan moving pattern belongs to Water in the Five Phases. The Qi circulates like water flowing in a curved river: smooth, and reaching every tiny area. When the Qi circulation can be smooth and harmonious, the Qi in the kidneys can be regulated. In addition, practicing Zuan can raise the clean Qi and sink the dirty Qi.

The documents have two sections and two songs which discuss Zuan Quan.

Figure 4-17

Figure 4-18

About Zuan Quan #1 鑽拳說一

Zuan Quan belongs to Water. The transportation of its Qi is like flowing water, smooth and curved, nowhere cannot be reached. Inside the body, it belongs to the kidneys, and in the fist it is Zuan. (If) it is performed correctly, then the Qi will be harmonious and the kidney('s Qi) sufficient. On the contrary, then the Qi is weird and the kidney('s Qi) deficient. (If) the Qi is weird and kidneys are void, then the clean Qi cannot be raised and the dirty Qi cannot be sunk. Furthermore, the real Jin of the fist will not be emitted. The practitioner should know about this.

鑽拳屬水，其氣之行，如水之委宛曲折，無不流到也。
在腹內則屬腎，在拳即為鑽。演之而合法，則氣和而腎
足，反之則氣乖而腎虛。氣乖腎虛，則清氣不能上升，
濁氣不能下降，而拳之真勁，亦不能出矣。學者當知之。

When Zuan Quan is performed it is like water which can flow everywhere. When the external motion is smooth, the Qi circulating in the body will also be like water flowing in a stream. Zuan Quan is related to the kidneys, which control the water in the body and are responsible for the moisture balance in the body. When your body is properly moisturized there will not be too much Fire (i.e., too much Yang), the clean Qi can be raised, and the dirty Qi can be sunk. This allows the mind to be calm and the body's Yin and Yang to be balanced.

From the point of view of Qigong, the motions of Zuan Quan alternately tenses and relaxes the back muscles, which massages the kidneys and smooths the Qi circulation.

About Zuan Quan #2 鑽拳說二

The shape of Zuan Quan is like thunder and its characteristics belong to Water. (If) it is discussed according to the theory of mutual production, Water is able to grow Wood, therefore, Zuan Quan is able to generate Beng Quan. (If) it is discussed from the theory of mutual conquest, Water is able to conquer Fire, therefore, Zuan Quan is able to conquer Pao Quan. When it is discussed according to the external manifestation of the Five Phases, the ears are connected to the kidneys. All of the above is the theory of mutual production and conquest of the Five Phases and also the theory of Zuan Quan.

鑽拳之形似雷電，性屬水。以相生之理論之，水能生木，
故鑽拳能生弸拳。以相克之理論之，水能克火，故鑽拳
能克炮拳。以五行隱於內者言，腎屬水。以五行著於外
者言，耳能通腎。此五行生克之理，鑽拳學之說也。

The motion of Zuan Quan, although smooth, is fast like thunder. In the theory of the Five Phases, Water is able to grow Wood and conquer Fire. Since Beng Quan belongs to Wood and relates to the liver in the Five Phases, Zuan Quan is able to generate Beng Quan. For the same reason, Pao Quan belongs to Fire and relates to the heart in the Five Phases, and Zuan Quan is able to conquer Pao Quan. In Chinese medicine, it is believed that the ears (which are shaped like kidneys) reflect the condition of the internal kidneys.

Zuan Quan Song #1 鑽拳歌一

The front Yin palm is holding downward and the rear Yang hand is drilling upward. The emitting hand drills up as high as the eyebrows. The two elbows are embracing the heart while moving the rear foot.

前手陰掌向下扣，後手陽拳往上鑽。
出拳高鑽如眉齊，兩肘抱心後腳起。

This section of the song describes the movements of Zuan Quan. When you per-form Zuan Quan the front hand is grabbing down with the palm facing down (Yin palm), while the rear hand is a fist drilling up and forward to the height of the eye-brows. Both elbows are dropped as if you were embracing your heart to protect your sides and the center of your chest. When executing Zuan Quan one leg steps forward and the other leg follows.

The eyes stare at the front fist and (the Qi) stops on (i.e., reaches to) the four extremities. (When) Zuan Quan is exchanging the postures, the body moves. The front foot steps first and the rear foot follows. The rear hand is a Yin palm and hides under the elbow.

眼看前拳四梢停，鑽拳換式身法動。
前腳先步後腳隨，後手陰掌肘下藏。

The eyes are looking forward and the Yi is concentrated. Use your Yi to lead the Qi to the four extremities (Si Shao, 四梢)(tongue, teeth, nails, and hair). When you do Zuan Quan ("exchange the postures"), one arm moves, and the leg on the same side of the body steps forward; then the other arm moves, and that leg follows. The rear hand is under the elbow of the front arm, palm facing down.

(Whenever) a step falls, the three tips must be aligned. The front hand is formed as a Yang fist and strikes the tip of the nose. The little finger is turned upward and the elbow is protecting the heart. (In) Zuan Quan, step forward and strike the tip of the nose. The front palm is holding (grabbing) the (opponent's) wrist and does Heng downward (and sideways). Step forward and turn the palm strike, striking the tiger relies on this.

落步總要三尖對，前手陽拳打鼻尖。
小指翻上肘護心，鑽拳進步打鼻尖。
前掌扣腕望下橫，進步掌翻打虎托。

The three tips should be lined up every time a foot hits the ground. The front hand is a fist with the palm facing up (Yang fist), and it is aiming for the opponent's nose. When you are doing the Yang fist, it is twisted so that the little finger is on top in order to generate a drilling motion. While you are striking with one hand, the other is holding or grabbing the opponent's wrist and pulling it strongly downward and to the side (i.e., Heng, 橫).

Zuan Quan Song #2 鑽拳歌二

Zuan Quan is like thunder and its characteristics belongs to Water. (It) produces Beng and conquers Pao, (you must use) the hands, feet, and legs. Raise for Zuan and fall for turning to turn around the Yin and Yang. (Its) ultimate achievement is to return to nothingness and wash the marrow/brain.

Figure 4-19

Figure 4-20

鑽拳似電性屬水，生弸克炮手足腿。
起鑽落翻陰陽轉，功至還虛是洗髓。

When Zuan Quan is raised for attack it is Yang, and when it falls it is Yin and you turn the foot and step forward to prepare for the next strike. The kidneys are considered the residence of Original Essence (Yuan Jing, 元精), which produces Water Qi. When this Qi is led to the brain for nourishment, it is able to wash the marrow and the brain and also raise up the spirit and lead it into the high domain of nothingness.

4.4.1 The Movements of Zuan Quan:

Right Hand Zuan:

1. Step into the three body posture (Figure 4-19).

2. Bring the left hand back to the waist, both hands form fists in front of your abdomen with palms down. Step forward with the left leg and at the same time drill the left fist from the waist up and forward (Figure 4-20).

3. The right leg steps forward and the left leg follows. While your are stepping, pull your left hand down to your abdomen (palm facing down) while

Figure 4-21

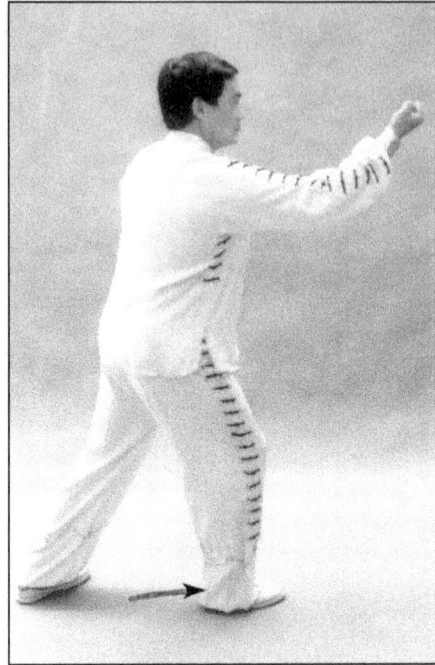
Figure 4-22

drilling the right fist up and forward toward the opponent's nose. At the conclusion of the technique, shift 60% of your weight to your rear leg (Figure 4-21).

Left Hand Zuan:

4. From the last posture, step your right leg forward (Figure 4-22).

5. Then step your left leg forward while the right leg follows. While you are stepping, pull your right hand down to the abdomen (palm down) and at the same time drill your left hand up and forward to attack the opponent's nose area. At the conclusion of the technique, shift 60% of your weight to your rear leg (Figure 4-23).

Figure 4-23

Figure 4-24

Changing Direction:

6. If you are in left Zuan, pivot your left foot and shift your weight onto it, and turn your body clockwise (Figure 4-24).

7. Finally, your right leg steps forward and the left leg follows. While you are stepping, pull your left hand back to your abdomen and at the same time drill your right fist forward and upward toward the opponent's nose (Figure 4-25).

Figure 4-25

Application of Zuan Quan:

When your opponent punches you with his right fist, cover it down with your left hand (Figure 4-26) and immediately step forward with your left leg (the right leg follows). While you are stepping, use the forward momentum to drill your right fist upward and forward to the opponent's face (Figure 4-27).

Figure 4-26

4.5 BENG QUAN

The Chinese word "Beng" (弸) means to stretch, develop, extend, and expand powerfully. It feels like a strong bow which has been drawn, and whose power is able to crush anything. In Xingyiquan, the Beng moving pattern belongs to Wood in the Five Phases. It is like a tree which can grow and be bent like a bow. The Qi in this pattern extends and

Figure 4-27

withdraws. When the Beng movement is smooth it can benefit the Qi circulation in the liver. Furthermore, this movement can raise the spirit of vitality, strengthen the physical body, and supply plenty of Qi nourishment to the brain.

There are two sections and two songs which describe Beng Quan in the documents.

About Beng Quan #1 崩拳說一

Beng Quan belongs to Wood. The to and fro of the two hands (i.e., emitting and withdrawing) is like arrows shooting continuously. This is the extending and withdrawing of the Qi. In the body it belongs to the liver, and when manifested externally it is Beng (Quan). If it is performed correctly, then the Qi can be peaceful, make the liver comfortable, raise up the spirit of vitality, strengthen the tendons and bones, and enhance brain power. Its benefits are not shallow.

崩拳屬木，兩手之往來，似箭出連珠，蓋一氣之伸縮也。
在腹內則屬肝，在拳即為崩。若演得其法，則能平氣舒
肝，長精神，強筋骨，壯腦力，為益非淺鮮也。

When Beng Quan is performed, it is like arrows shot from a bow. The Qi in the body feels like it is extending as far as an arrow can reach. When the Jin is stored, it is like the bow is bent and ready to shoot. Beng Quan belongs to Wood and corresponds to the liver. From the Qigong point of view, the motion of Beng Quan is able to regulate the Qi in the liver. In addition, practicing Beng Quan can raise the spirit and strengthen the tendons and bones. According to Qigong, the liver relates to the soul or the spirit of the body, and is connected to the eyes.

About Beng Quan #2 崩拳說二

The shape of Beng Quan is like an arrow and its characteristics belong to Wood. Discussing it according to the theory of mutual production, Wood is able to produce Fire, therefore Beng Quan is able to generate Pao Quan. Discussing it according to the theory of mutual conquest, Wood is able to conquer Earth, and therefore Beng Quan is able to conquer Heng Quan. (If) discussing it according to the Five Phases which are hidden internally, the liver belongs to Wood. (If) discussing it according to the Five Phases which are manifesting externally, the eyes are connected to the liver. This is the theory of mutual production and conquest in the Five Phases. (It is also) the theory of Beng Quan.

崩拳之形似箭，性屬木。由相生之理論之，木能生火，
故崩拳能生炮拳。由相克之理論之，木能克土，故崩拳
能克橫拳。以五行隱於內者言，肝屬水。以五行著於外
者言，目能通肝。此五行生克之理，崩拳學之說也。

Beng Quan belongs to Wood in the Five Phases and relates to the liver. Therefore, it is able to generate Fire and conquer Earth. In Xingyiquan, since Pao Quan belongs to Fire and Heng Quan belongs to Earth, Beng Quan is able to generate Pao Quan and conquer Heng Quan. Chinese medicine believes that the eyes reveal and manifest the spirit, and refer to this as the "Yan Shen" (眼神), or "eye spirit."

In addition, the spirit of the eyes shows the condition of the liver. If you tire very easily your eyes will not be bright and shiny. This usually implies that the liver is in poor condition.

Beng Quan Song #1 弸拳歌一

When the Beng Quan posture is emitted, the three tips are lined up. The tiger eye (of the striking hand) is facing upward and is as the high as the heart. The rear hand forms the Yang fist and is hidden under the armpit. The front foot must (move) smoothly and the rear foot form a word Ding (the letter T).

弸拳出勢三尖對，虎眼朝上如心齊。
後手陽拳脅下藏，前腳要順後腳丁。

When Beng Quan is performed, the tips of the hands, feet, and nose should line up. The tiger's eye of the striking hand is facing upward and strikes as high as the solar plexus. The tiger's eye is the hole which is formed in the tiger's mouth area when the hand is closed in a fist. While you are striking, the rear fist is palm up on the abdomen under the elbow of the front hand (Yang fist). When you are striking, the movement of the front foot should be smooth and the rear foot follows to form the letter T. When you are striking with Beng Quan, the forward Jin is supported by the rear foot. A correct stance will support and enhance the manifestation of Beng Jin.

In order to be steady on the rear foot, (the feet) must form the shape of (the word) man. (When) performing Beng Quan and turning the body, (the hand is) as high as the eyebrows. The body is standing upright while raising the foot. The foot is raised under the knee and the toes are sideways.

後腳穩要人字形，弸拳翻身望眉齊。
身站正直腳提起，腳起膝下橫腳趾。

This section of the song discusses how to position the feet in order to be steady and make the Jin powerful. The two feet should form an upside-down V, like the Chinese word for man. In order to do this, the front toes should be slightly inward while the toes of the rear foot face 45 degree to the side. When stepping, the body should always be upright.

The foot and the hands fall together and the thighs are like scissors. The front foot must step with Heng and the rear foot follows smoothly. The way of striking in Beng Quan is the tip of tongue presses upward. In the front arm, the elbow is pulled and (the fist) is pressed upward. When you step forward and emit the fist, first strike the flank. The rear foot is tightly connected and follows.

腳手齊落剪子股，前腳要橫後腳順。
彆拳打法舌尖頂，前手攔肘望上托。
進步出拳先打脅，後腳是連緊隨跟。

In Beng Quan, the hands and rear foot all fall together. In order to make the stance firm and strong to support the Jin, the thighs move like a pair of scissors. When you move, the front leg moves with a forceful, sideward power to open the way while the rear foot follows smoothly. The tongue is pressed gently to the roof of the mouth. The elbow of the striking hand should be dropped and the striking power is forward and upward at the level of the armpit. You can see from this song that Beng Quan strikes three places: the solar plexus, the face (eyebrow), and the flank.

Beng Quan Song #2 彆拳歌二

Beng Quan is like an arrow and its characteristics belong to Wood. (It) produces Pao and conquers Heng, this theory is not ridiculous. The two fists advance in turn and continuously. Remember firmly that the left (leg) is in front, and the right foot is in the rear.

彆拳似箭性屬木，生炮克橫理不謬。
兩拳輪流循環進，牢記左前右足後。

Traditionally, when you do Beng Quan the left foot is always forward. The front leg moves first and the rear foot follows tightly. While you are moving your feet, the two fists continue to strike with the support of the rear leg.

4.5.1 The Movements of Beng Quan:

Right Hand Beng:

1. Step into the three body posture (Figure 4-28).
2. Make fists with both hands, while turning the body clockwise slightly (Figure 4-29).
3. Step forward with the left leg, pull the left fist back to your waist with the palm facing up while punching the right fist forward with the tiger eye facing upward. While you are punching, you also take a small step forward with your right leg to follow the left leg (Figure 4-30). The right foot should stamp the ground at the same time as you punch in order to bounce the power from the ground to support the punch. Then shift 60% of your weight to your rear leg.

Figure 4-28

Figure 4-29

Left Hand Beng:

4. Step forward with the left leg and punch forward with the left hand while the right hand pulls back to the waist. The right leg follows the left and steps forward and stamps the floor just as the punch hits to support it, and then you shift 60% of your weight to it (Figure 4-31).

Changing Direction:

5. When you run out of space and your left Beng is forward, pivot your left foot and shift all of your weight to it, turn your body clockwise and at the same time bring the left fist to your waist. The palms of both fists should face upward (Figure 4-32).

6. Drill the right fist up from the waist and at the same time kick out with the right heel about knee level (Figure 4-33).

Figure 4-30

Figure 4-31

Figure 4-32

Figure 4-33

Figure 4-34

Figure 4-35

7. Step your right foot down and turn your body clockwise into the posture of "Sitting with Crossed Legs" (Zuo Pan Bu, 坐盤步). While you are doing this, your hands are performing Left Pi (Figure 4-34).

8. Make fists with both hands (Figure 4-35).

9. Step forward with the left foot and punch with the right fist while the left fist pulls back to the waist and at the same time the right leg steps forward and stamps the floor (Figure 4-36).

Figure 4-36

Application of Beng Quan:

When your opponent punches you with his right fist, simply use your left hand to direct his punch down as you step your left leg forward (Figure 4-37). Your right leg follows, hitting the ground to bounce the right Beng into the opponent's solar plexus area (Figure 4-38).

Figure 4-37

Figure 4-38

4.6 PAO QUAN

The Chinese word "Pao" (炮) has the sense of an explosion, like a cannon shooting a cannonball. The power is straight forward, strong, fast, and destructive. In the Five Phases, the Pao moving pattern belongs to Fire, and is related to the heart. In the Pao movement, the Qi either is closed and remains quiet, or bursts open like an explosion, fast and powerful. When the Pao movement is smooth, the stagnant Qi stored in the body can be released and emitted from the body. This movement will help release the Fire accumulated in the heart and make the body feel comfortable.

About Pao Quan #1 炮拳說一

Pao Quan belongs to Fire and is the opening and closing of the one Qi. Like a cannon suddenly blasting and suddenly hurling its ball. Its nature is the most violent and its shape (i.e., appearance) is the most fiery. In the body, it belongs to the heart, and in the fist, it is Pao. (If) it is performed correctly, then the body is comfortable and unrestrained, and the Qi is harmonized. (If) it is performed incorrectly, then (the movements of) the four limbs are not smooth and the Qi is weird. When its Qi is harmonious, then inside the heart is clear and spiritual. When its Qi is weak, then inside the heart is blurred and confused. The learner should study deeply.

炮拳屬火，是一氣之開合，如炮忽然炸裂，其彈突出，其性最烈，其形最猛。在腹內則屬心，在拳則為炮。演之合法，則身體舒暢而氣和；演之不合，則四體不順而氣乖。其氣和，則心中虛靈，其氣乖，則心中朦昧。學者當深究之。

When Pao Quan is performed it is like a cannon firing. When its Jin is manifested the stagnant Qi in the heart can be released to the surface of the body. Therefore, if you do it correctly, you will be able to regulate the heart Qi and also make the Jin powerful like a cannon. The heart is also related to your emotions. If the Qi is circulating smoothly in the heart, your emotions will be clear and the spirit can be raised high. However, if there is some Qi stagnation in your heart, then your emotions will not be clear and you will be confused.

About Pao Quan #2 炮拳說二

The shape of Pao Quan is like a cannon firing, its characteristics belong to Fire. When it is applied in the theory of mutual production, Fire is able to produce Earth. Therefore, Pao Quan is able to produce Heng Quan. When it is applied in the theory of mutual conquest, Fire is able to conquer Metal. Therefore, Pao Quan is able to conquer Pi Quan. When it is applied in the Five Phases which are hidden internally, the Heart belongs to Fire. When it is used in the Five Phas-

es which are manifested externally, the tongue is able to communicate with the heart. This is the theory of mutual production and conquest in the Five Phases and it is also the theory of Pao Quan. Pao Quan is number four of the five fists, however, it is slightly harder than the other four fists to practice. Because if there is any misunderstanding, then it is not easy to understand the Jin.

炮拳之形似炮，性屬火。由相生之理論之，火能生土，
故炮拳能生橫拳。以相克之理論之，火能克金，故炮拳
能克劈拳。以五行隱於內者言，心屬火。以五行著於外
者言，舌能通心。此五行生克之理，炮拳學之說也。炮
拳為五行拳之四，然練習較五行中之餘四拳稍為困難。
因偶一背謬，即不易懂勁故耳。

Pao Quan belongs to Fire and relates to the heart in the Five Phases. In the Five Phases, Fire is able to produce Earth and conquer Metal, therefore Pao Quan can produce Heng Quan and conquer Pi Quan. It is believed that the tongue is related to the heart, so you are able to understand the condition of the heart from the condition of the tongue. Although the movements of Pao Quan are not difficult, its deeper meaning is the hardest to understand. In order to make the Pao Jin strong, the emotional mind must be stimulated to a high level, and this emotional feeling is then exploded into the Jin.

Song of Pao Quan #1　炮拳歌一

Two elbows embrace tightly and raise up the feet. Two fists are tightened and the Yang fists are required. The front hand must be Heng and the rear arm bent. Two fists are as high as embracing the navel.

兩肘緊抱腳提起，兩拳一緊要陽拳。
前手要橫後手丁，兩拳高只肚臍抱。

When you start the Pao Quan movement, sink your elbows and keep them in tight to protect your chest. The hands are Yang fists, with the palms facing sideward (palm up or sideward is Yang, palm facing down in Yin). The front arm is used for blocking and clearing the way to the side. The rear arm is not straightened out completely when it punches. When you prepare for an attack, the hands are in front of the navel.

Qi follows the body movement and enters the Dan Tian. The hands and feet fall together and the three tips line up. (When) the fist strikes, it is only as high as the heart. The tiger's eye of the front hand is facing upward.

氣就身法入丹田，腳手齊落三尖對。
拳打高只與心齊，前拳虎眼朝上頂。

Qi follows the motions of the body, so when you bring your arms in at the beginning of the movement, Qi also condenses, and accumulates in the Dan Tian. When you strike, the tips of your lead foot, punching hand, and your nose should be in the same plane. When striking, the striking area should only be as high as the solar plexus. Because the heart is well protected by the ribs, Chinese martial arts traditionally attack it by way of the solar plexus. The solar plexus is called "Xin Wo" (心窩), which means "heart cave" or "heart entrance." The tiger's eye of the punching hand faces up.

The rear fist drills upward to the eyebrows. The eye of the tiger is facing downward and the elbow is dropped. (When) Pao Quan (begins to) strike, the (front) foot is raised. (As) the step falls, the front fist drills upward. Fists and feet fall together with crossing step. The rear leg follows closely with Heng.

後拳上鑽眉上齊，虎眼朝下肘下垂。
炮拳打法腳提起，落步前拳望上鑽。
拳腳齊落十字步，後腳是連緊隨橫。

The blocking fist drills upward to the height of the eyebrows. The palm of the fist is turned outward, the tiger's eye is facing downward, and the elbow is dropped. When you strike with Pao Quan, step forward with the Heng force and the rear leg naturally follows.

Song of Pao Quan #2 炮拳歌二

Pao Quan is like a cannon firing, and its characteristics belong to Fire. (It) produces Heng (Quan) and conquer Pi (Quan), combining the internal and external. There is no problem if you move diagonally and follow the fighting strategy. Understand the essence and the meaning of the five fists and thirteen rules.

炮拳似炮性屬火，生橫克劈內外合。
斜行何妨從軍陣，五拳精義十三格。

It is believed that the explosive Jin of Pao Quan is able to release internal stagnation out of the body. Normally, the front hand and leg use Heng Jin to force the way in and clear the way for the strike. If you are able to comprehend the deep meaning of Pao Quan, you will be able to grasp the keys to the Jins of the five fists and really understand the rules described in the second chapter.

Figure 4-39

Figure 4-40

4.6.1 Movements of Pao Quan:

Right Hand Pao:

1. Step into the three body posture (Figure 4-39).

2. Step forward and slightly to the side with the left leg as you stretch out your hands with the palms facing each other (Figure 4-40).

3. Move the right foot up to the left foot and parallel to it, and at the same time make a grabbing motion with both hands and bring them in and down to the waist. Close your hands into fists as you bring them in and face them upward (Figure 4-41).

Figure 4-41

Figure 4-42

Figure 4-43

4. Step 45 degrees to the left with the left foot, block up with the left arm and punch with the right fist while taking a step forward with the right foot and hitting the floor to bounce the Jin upward from the foot. Finally, shift 60% of your weight to your rear leg (Figure 4-42).

Left Hand Pao:

5. Step out with your left leg and reach out with your open hands as in Figure 4-40. Move the right foot parallel to the left foot and bring both fists to the waists with palms facing up (Figure 4-43).

6. Step your right leg 45 degrees to the right, block with the right arm and punch with the left fist while the left leg follows and stamps the floor as described above (Figure 4-44).

Figure 4-44

Figure 4-45

Figure 4-46

Changing Direction:

7. If you have just done left Pao and have run out of space, turn your body to your left and step your right leg to the outside of your left leg. Shift your weight to your right leg and let your left foot pivot so that it is facing the same direction as your body. As you turn your body, bring both fists to your waist with the palms facing up (Figure 4-45). Then step your left leg forward and slightly to the side for right hand Pao as your right foot follows and stamps the floor (Figure 4-46).

Application of Pao Quan:

When your opponent punches with his fight fist, simply use your left hand to block his punch up and lead it to the side to seal his arm while you step to his right. While you are blocking, your right hand Pao strikes the opponent's chest or solar plexus (Figure 4-47).

Figure 4-47

4.7 HENG QUAN

The word "Heng" (横) means to cross, move sideways, or to force through aggressively with a sideward motion. It also has the sense of two forces moving in opposite directions to balance each other. In the Five Phases, this movement belongs to Earth, and is related to the spleen and the stomach. This movement is able to make the Qi gathered at its center (i.e., between the solar plexus and the navel)(Figure 4-48) round and full. When the Qi is smooth from doing the Heng movement, then the other four Qis will coordinate with each other harmoniously.

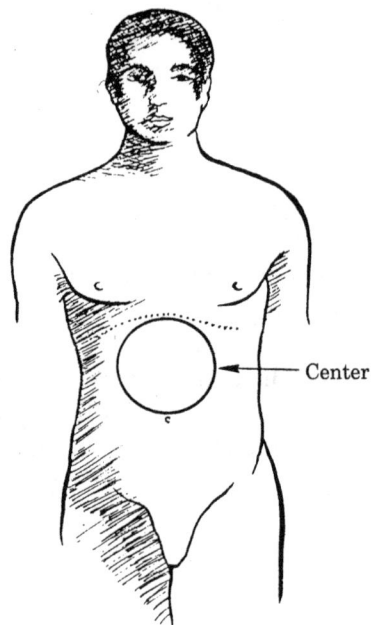

Figure 4-48. The "Center" of the body

About Heng Quan #1 橫拳說一

Heng Quan belongs to Earth and is the gathering of the one Qi. In the body, it belongs to the spleen and in the fist it is Heng. Its Qi must be smooth. When smooth, then the spleen and the stomach are peaceful and move slowly, otherwise, the spleen and stomach will be void and weak. In addition, its Quan (i.e., performance) must be accurate. When it is accurate, then the Five Phases are harmonious internally and hundreds of bodies are comfortable and expanded. Incorrect, then the internal Qi loses harmony and the movements will lose control. In all, its nature must be solid, the Qi smooth, the shape round, and the Jin coordinated (i.e., Qi and Li), then (you) will be able to fulfill the potential of Heng. The ancestors said: "On the theory (of mutual relations), it is trust. In man, it is in the spleen. In the fist, then it is Heng."

> 橫拳屬土，是一氣之團聚也。在腹內則屬脾，在拳則為橫。其氣要順，順則脾胃和緩，否則脾胃虛弱。又其拳要合式，合則內五行和而百體均舒暢。謬則內氣失和，而舉動咸失措。總要性實、氣順、形圓、勁和，方能盡橫拳之能事。先哲云：〝在理則為信，在人則為脾，在拳則屬橫〞是也。

Heng Quan belongs to Earth and relates to the spleen, which is considered to be neutral, or the center of the Five Phases. It is located centrally between Yin and Yang, and constitutes a bridge between them. Therefore, if the spleen Qi is harmonious, then the Yin and Yang can harmoniously cooperate and interact with each other. This is why it says that the spleen is like the trust in an interpersonal relationship, because it builds up the bridge of communication. In the body, spleen Qi acts as the connection between Yin and Yang. Therefore, in the Five Fists, Heng Quan is the center one which coordinates with the Yin and Yang strategy of the other four fists.

About Heng Quan #2 橫拳說二

The shape of Heng Quan is like a ball, its characteristics belong to Earth. When it is applied in the theory of mutual production, Earth is able to produce Metal. Therefore, Heng Quan is able to produce Pi Quan. When it is applied in the theory of mutual conquest, Earth is able to conquer Water. Therefore, Heng Quan is able to conquer Zuan Quan. When it is applied in the Five Phases which are hidden internally, the Spleen belongs to Earth. When it is used in the Five Phases which are manifested externally, Renzhong is able to communicate with the Spleen. This is the theory of mutual production and conquest in the Five Phases, and it is also the theory of Heng Quan.

> 橫拳之形似彈，性屬土。以相生之理論之，土能生金，故橫拳能生劈拳。以相克之理論之，土能克水，故橫拳能克鑽拳。以五行隱於內者言，脾屬土。以五行著於外者言，人中能通脾。此五行生克之理，橫拳學之說也。

Heng Quan is a sideward strike and moves with a rounded motion. It is round like the earth and neutral like the earth. In the Five Phases, Earth is able to produce Metal and conquer Water. Therefore, in the five fists, Heng Quan can produce Pi Quan and conquer Zuan Quan. Renzhong (Gv-26)(人中) is the cavity located between the nose and upper lip. It is related to the spleen, and reflects the condition of the spleen.

Song of Heng Quan #1　橫拳歌一

The front hand is Yang Quan and the rear is Yin. The rear hand is always hiding under the armpit. (When I) exchange the posture and release my hand (i.e., attack), the leg raises (for action). (When I) stand still, the Qi is able to transport.

前手陽拳後手陰，後手只在脅下藏。
換式出手腳提起，身法一站氣能通。

When you perform Heng Quan, the palm of the front fist faces up (Yang fist) and the palm of the rear fist faces down (Yin fist). The rear fist is always hidden at your side. When you start the move, your rear leg starts to step forward and your hands begin to exchange their positions. When you stand still, the mind is clear and the Qi is unrestrained.

The tongue curves upward and Qi is emitted. (When) Heng Quan is changing the postures, the thighs are like scissors. Triangular body; moving the important stepping, feet and legs are maneuvered cleanly. (When) the rear hand is turning and becoming Yang, (it) repels toward the outside.

舌尖上捲氣外發，橫拳換式剪子股。
斜身要步腳手落，後手翻陽望外撥。

The tongue is touching the roof of the mouth to connect the Yin and Yang vessels (Conception and Governing Vessels)(任脈、督脈). This makes it possible for the Qi to circulate smoothly and abundantly and energize the muscles so that your Jin can be efficient. When you do Heng, keep your thighs close together to protect your groin and strengthen your stance. As you step, the thighs pass close by each other like the two halves of a scissors. Keep your body turned to the side (triangular) to minimize the area exposed to your opponent. As your rear hand moves to strike, it turns palm up (Yang fist) and moves to the side.

When the step falls, the three tips of Yang Quan match each other. The tip of the nose and the tip of the foot should be closely connected. (When) Heng Quan is used for striking, the rear fist is Yin. The front hand is Yang Quan and its elbow protects the heart. Left and right bend the bow and repel to the outside. The feet and hands fall at the same time and the tongue tip is curved.

落步陽拳三尖對，鼻尖腳尖緊相連。
橫拳打法後拳陰，前手陽拳肘護心。
左右開弓望外撥，腳手齊落舌尖捲。

When you step down, the three tips should be lined up. When you repel the opponent's force to the side, it is like you are bending a bow to the side, strongly and forcefully When performing Heng Quan, you move one arm forward and to the side, while the other arm moves downward to the side to balance the motion.

Song of Heng Quan #2　橫拳歌二

Heng Quan (moves) like a ball and its characteristics belong to Earth. (It) produces Pi (Quan) and conquers Zuan (Quan), the movements must be sure to match the curve. Hook (i.e., twist) the thighs and become triangular at the very hidden place. Heart, Liver, Spleen, Lungs, and Kidneys, (Heng) is the master.

橫拳似彈性屬土，生劈克鑽切合弧。
勾股三角極微處，心肝脾胃腎為主。

Heng Quan is able to produce Pi Quan and conquer Zuan Quan. The movements are curved. The key to stability is keeping the thighs close together and the hips turned. This also protects the groin (the "very hidden place"). Heng is the center of the five fists and coordinates the other four. It is therefore the master key of the five fists.

4.7.1 Movements of Heng Quan:

Right Hand Heng:

1. Step into the three body posture (Figure 4-49).

2. The left foot takes a step forward and slightly to the side, both hands close into fists, the right hand with the palm up goes underneath the left arm and then thrusts up and to the front and right, while the left hand with the palm down pulls down and back to the right elbow. At the same

Figure 4-49

Figure 4-50

Figure 4-51

time the right foot takes a small step forward and stamps (Figure 4-50). Strike with the middle knuckle of the index finger, and shift 60% of your weight to your rear leg at the conclusion of the technique.

Left Hand Heng:

3. The left foot steps forward with a small step, the right foot slides next to the left foot then forward to the right. While you are stepping, turn the left palm face up and move it underneath the right arm forward and to the left, while the right fist turns palm down and retracts next to the left elbow. When you strike with the left hand, the left foot stamps on the ground to generate the bouncing Jin to support the strike. Shift 60% of your weight to your rear leg at the conclusion of the technique (Figure 4-51).

Figure 4-52

Figure 4-53

Changing Direction:

4. If you have just done a left Heng, pivot your right foot and shift your weight onto it, and turn your body counterclockwise (Figure 4-52).

5. Take a step forward with the left leg, strike with right Heng and pull back the left hand (Figure 4-53).

4.7.2 Application of Heng Quan:

When your opponent punches with his right fist, intercept it with your left hand and circle it to the side while at the same time stepping to his right and striking him from the side with your right fist (Figure 4-54).

Figure 4-54

Five Phases Linking Sequence 五行連環拳

5.1 INTRODUCTION

In this chapter we will introduce the most important and most basic sequence or practice routine in Xingyiquan: the Five Phases Linking Sequence (Wu Xing Lian Huan Quan, 五行連環拳). This sequence is constructed from the five basic fists (moving patterns) introduced in Chapter 4. As you learn this sequence you are like a baby learning how to walk. You are beginning to gradually grasp the keys and tricks of Xingyiquan. You are learning about the unique essence of this style, and what distinguishes it from all other internal styles. There are a few general points which we would like to make about the purpose of training this sequence.

1. It links and combines the five fists, and you learn to master the five fists through repeated practice.

2. You begin to understand the theory of mutual production and conquest and apply it in the applications.

3. You begin to understand the basic requirements of Xingyiquan, which reveal its essence. The art has taken these and built up its own unique theory and applications in both martial arts and health.

4. You learn to unify the external manifestation (shape) and the internal mind (Yi), and from this unification to build the Qi to a higher level and circulate it smoothly. Through this unification you also learn how to raise up your spirit of vitality. Remember, the internal is Yin and the external is Yang, and only if you can combine them harmoniously will you be able to grasp the essence of Xingyiquan.

5. You train the five basic Jins in the five fists, which teaches you how to apply the Qi in the movements to energize the muscles to their maximum efficiency.

There is a song which talks about the Five Phases Linking Sequence:

Song of the Linking Sequence 連環拳歌

Quickly advance and quickly withdraw, the postures are linked and threaded. Suddenly short and suddenly long, its meaning and theory are detailed (i.e., clear). (It) combines the one Qi and its domain is vast. Move repeatedly left and right as if you were next to a wall.

倏進倏退式連環，忽短忽長義理詳。

混合一氣範圍廣，循環左右若傍牆。

In the Five Phases Linking Sequence you learn how to advance and retreat smoothly and naturally, so your attack can be long or short. All of the theory is detailed clearly in the applications. When you know how to combine and thread the random Qi into one Qi, you will be able to act with your Qi body and physical body as one. Then the applications of this one Qi will be boundless. Repeatedly move to the right and left as if you had forced your opponent against a wall.

5.2 MUTUAL PRODUCTION AND CONQUEST IN XINGYIQUAN

Chapter 4 has given you some basic concepts of the Five Fists or Five Phases of Xingyiquan. One of the most important aspects of these Five Fists is the relationship between them which is based on the theory of mutual production and conquest of the Five Phases. This theory is one of the most basic contents in the *Yi Jing* (易經) (*Book of Changes*). In this section we would first like to introduce several songs about these relationships.

Song of Mutual Production 相生歌

Pi is able to generate Zuan and Zuan is able to produce Beng. Beng is capable of bearing Pao and Pao is able to beget Heng. Heng is able to move into Pi, each one manifests its unique essence. The millions of lives returning to the dust is caused by these Five Phases.

劈能生鑽鑽生弸，弸能生炮炮生橫。

橫能生劈各形本，萬物於土五行生。

In Xingyiquan, Pi (劈) is Metal (Jin, 金), Zuan (鑽) is Water (Shui, 水), Beng (弸) is Wood (Mu, 木), Pao (炮) is Fire (Huo, 火), and Heng (橫) is Earth (or dust)(Tu, 土). According to the theory of mutual production and conquest in the Five Phases (Wu Xing, 五行), Metal is able to generate Water, Water is able to grow Wood, Wood is able to generate Fire, Fire results in the production of ashes (Earth), and finally, Earth produces Metal (Figure 5-1).

When these relationships are applied to Xingyiquan, you may see clearly that in the fighting strategy of Xingyiquan, Pi Quan can be followed by Zuan Quan. Zuan

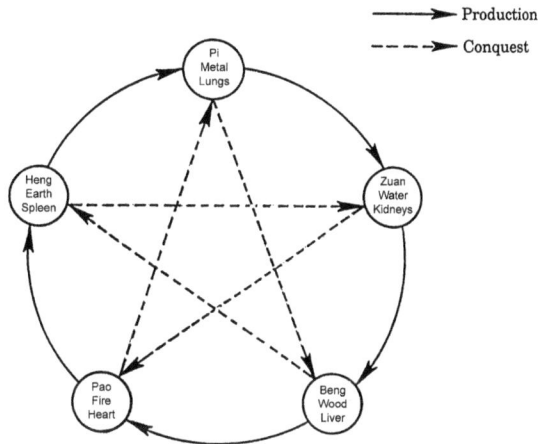

Figure 5-1. The relationships between the Five Phases

Quan is able to move into Beng Quan, and Beng Quan can produce Pao Quan. Pao Quan can be followed by Heng Quan, and finally, Heng Quan can be followed by Pi Quan.

The last sentence in the text says that it does not matter which Fist you are applying, Heng (Earth) is always the center of the Five Phases. The earth (or dust) is the origin of all life, and its final resting place. In the same way, Heng is the foundation of the other four Fists, and they are all built upon Heng. For example, Pi needs Heng, Zuan needs Heng, Beng needs Heng, and Pao also needs Heng. Heng is not used only to clear the way for an attack, it can also be used to attack in the same way as you would force your way in. Therefore, in the Five Fists, Heng is the root and the center of the other four Fists.

You can see that the offensive applications of the Five Fists are linked together through these relationships of production and conquest. The Five Phases Linking Sequence was created to help the beginner understand the Five Phases theory in Xingyiquan. Therefore, you should not only learn the forms of the Linking Sequence in this chapter, but also study the theory and try to really comprehend its essence.

Song of Mutual Conquest 相克歌

Pi is able to conquer Beng and Beng is able to defeat Heng. Heng is able to subjugate Zuan and Zuan is able to overmaster Pao. Pao can overcome Pi, (all of these are) belong to the theory of Yi (Yi Jing, The Book of Change). Looking for the real meaning is nowhere else but within the Five Phases.

劈能克弸弸克橫，橫能克鑽鑽克炮。
炮能克劈歸易理，不外五行求真諦。

Figure 5-2

Figure 5-3

The theory of mutual conquest establishes the relationships of defense in the Five Fists (Figure 5-1). Pi can be used against Beng, Beng is able to upset Heng, Heng is able to defeat Zuan, Zuan can be used to defend against Pao, and finally Pao has the ability to overcome Pi.

The best way to practice the actions of this theory is to practice them repeatedly with a partner. This is the reason for the creation of the fighting set An Shen Pao (安身炮)(Secure Body Strike), which will be discussed in Chapter 7.

5.3 FIVE PHASES LINKING SEQUENCE

We have discussed the basic level of martial applications of the Five Phases in Chapter 4, and so we will not repeat them here, but will only discuss the movements of the Five Phases Linking Sequence.

Five Phases Linking Sequence (Wu Xing Lian Huan Quan) 五行連環拳

1. Stand straight and look forward (Figure 5-2).

2. Turn your body slightly to the right and move into the three body posture (Figures 5-3 to 5-5).

3. Right hand Pi (Figures 5-6 to 5-8).

Figure 5-4

Figure 5-5

Figure 5-6

Figure 5-7

Figure 5-8

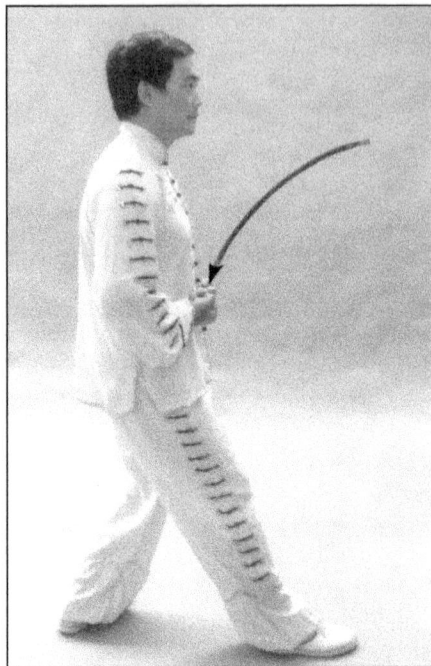

Figure 5-9

4. Left hand Pi (Figures 5-9 to 5-11).

5. Right hand Beng (Figures 5-12).

6. Step your right leg back with a small step (Figure 5-13) and bring the left leg behind the right leg into a sitting crossed legs stance. When you are stepping, punch your left fist forward while pulling your right fist back to the abdomen area (Figure 5-14).

Figure 5-10

Figure 5-11

Figure 5-12

Figure 5-13

Figure 5-14

Figure 5-15

Figure 5-16

7. Turn your body to the left and take a small step forward with the right leg, punch with the right hand and pull the left hand back to the waist while the left leg follows with a step forward and stamps to bounce the Jin upward (Figure 5-15).

8. Shift your weight to your left leg, and bring your right fist down and place it over your left hand (Figure 5-16).

9. Open both hands and spread them out to make a circle in front of your body as you shift your weight forward (Figure 5-17).

10. Bring back the right arm, hit the back of the right fist into the palm of the left hand and at the same time bring back the right foot and stamp (Figure 5-18).

11. Left hand Pao (Figure 5-19).

12. Bring the right leg back behind the left leg, pull the left hand back to the waist, and at the same time sweep your right forearm down past your face (Figure 5-20).

Figure 5-17

Figure 5-18

Figure 5-19

Figure 5-20

Figure 5-21

Figure 5-22

13. Sit back and place all of your weight on your right leg (Figure 5-21).

14. Then step your left leg forward for left hand Pi (Figure 5-22).

15. Step 30 degrees to the left with the left leg, the right arm does Zuan and the left fist pulls down next to your right elbow while the right foot slides up naturally. This and the following movement step to the side of the opponent, so although the leg steps to the corner, the punch still goes in the direction of your original line of advance (Figure 5-23).

16. Step 60 degrees to the right with the right leg, the left arm does Zuan and the right fist pulls down next to the left elbow while the left foot naturally slides up (Figure 5-24).

17. Step 45 degrees to the right of your line of advance with your right leg and reach out with both open hands, then place the left foot next to the right foot while pulling both hands to the waist (Figure 5-25).

18. Do Right Hand Pao to your left (Figure 5-26).

Figure 5-23

Figure 5-24

Figure 5-25

Figure 5-26

Figure 5-27

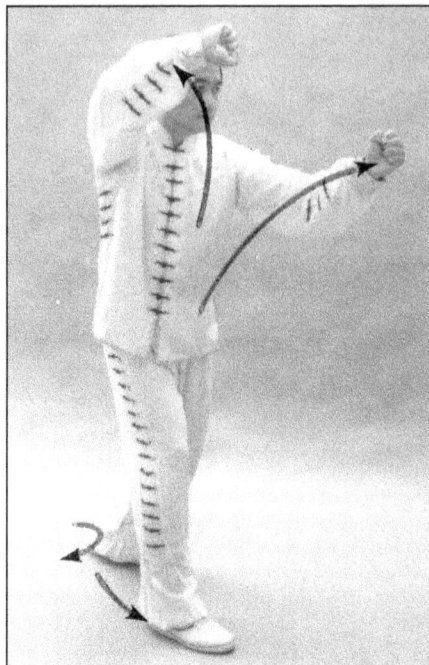

Figure 5-28

19. Step in the same direction with the left leg and reach out with both open hands, then place the right foot next to the left foot while pulling both hands to the waist (Figure 5-27).

20. Do Left Hand Pao to your right (Figure 5-28).

21. The right arm does Zuan and at the same time the right leg kicks (Figure 5-29).

22. Put the right leg down into a sitting on crossed legs stance while the arms do Left Hand Pi (Figure 5-30).

23. Step forward with your left leg for Right Hand Heng (Figure 5-31).

24. Step forward with your right leg for Left Hand Heng (Figure 5-32).

Figure 5-29

Figure 5-30

Figure 5-31

Figure 5-32

Figure 5-33

Figure 5-34

25. Open both hands and start circling them down and to your left. Pivot your right foot to the right as the arms circle up and in front of you. Step forward with your left foot as the left hand stretches out in front of you and the right hand comes in to your waist (Figure 5-33). Then do Right Hand Beng and follow with the right foot (Figure 5-34).

26. Pivot your left foot, shift your weight to it, and turn your whole body clockwise while the right hand is brought back to the waist (Figure 5-35).

27. The right arm does Zuan and the right leg kicks (Figure 5-36).

28. Place the right foot down in front and turn the body to get into a sitting on crossed legs stance while the arms do Left Hand Pi (Figure 5-37).

You may now repeat the sequence by stepping forward with your left leg and doing Right Hand Beng, and then continuing from Figure 5-12. You may repeat the sequence as many times as you wish. When you have reached Figure 5-37 and decide to stop, step your right leg back past your left leg and then bring your left leg back next to it, and at the same time bring your hands down to your sides (Figure 5-38).

Figure 5-35

Figure 5-36

Figure 5-37

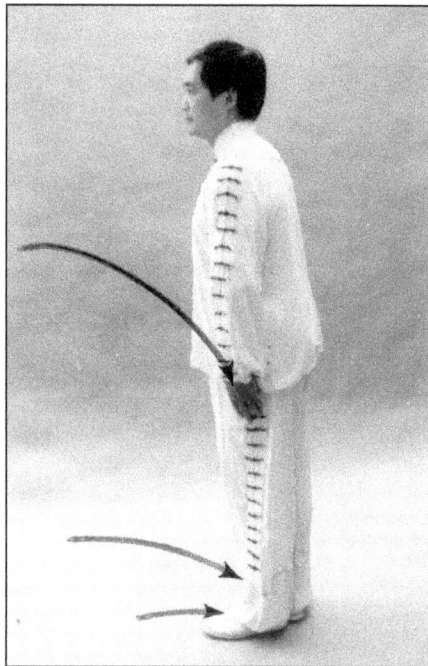

Figure 5-38

Xingyiquan 形意拳

6.1 INTRODUCTION

Once you have mastered the Five Phases Linking Sequence you will want to enter deeper into the field of Xingyiquan training. Usually the sequence of Twelve Shapes (Shi Er Xing, 十二形) is then practiced. This sequence imitates the movements and fighting mentalities of twelve animals. Quite frequently the five fists are mixed with the twelve animals to form many different sequences.

Since the Twelve Shapes sequence is available in many Xingyiquan books, we would like to introduce instead a combination of the five fists and the twelve animal shapes which was constructed by Master Liang's teacher Master Zheng, Huai-Xian (鄭懷賢), and which is simply called Xingyiquan. The purpose of this sequence is twofold. First it introduces the twelve animal forms, and second it offers a guideline to combining the five fists and the twelve forms. Practicing this sequence will open your mind to comprehend the deeper meaning of Xingyiquan. Through this effort you may someday be able to understand deeply enough to construct correct Xingyiquan sequences of your own.

In this chapter we will discuss not only the forms of the sequence, but also introduce some of the applications. As you may already suspect, it would be impossible to introduce all of the possible applications in a single book. Therefore, the applications introduced in this chapter will stay only on the surface level. The main purpose of this is to help you understand the basic applications of each form. Once you comprehend this sequence, continued practice will help you to discover the keys to other, deeper levels of applications.

In order to be clear on the directions you should be facing while doing the movements, the direction you are facing as you begin the sequence will be considered north. Therefore, the direction to your left is west, the right is east, etc. In the pictures showing the applications, you are the person in the white uniform.

Figure 6-1

Figure 6-2

6.2 XINGYIQUAN

6.2.1 Xingyiquan 形意拳

Beginning (Qi Shi): 起式

1. Stand straight with a calm mind (Figure 6-1).

2. Turn your body slightly to the right and circle both hands upward (Figure 6-2).

3. Continue the motion and bring both hands down to the front of the abdomen, closing them palms down into fists as they sink (Figure 6-3).

Three Body Posture (San Ti Shi): 三體式

4. While keeping your feet in place, turn your body to your left, and drill your right fist up to face level. The right palm faces up, and your left fist is palm down under your right elbow (Figure 6-4).

5. Step your left leg forward and form the three body posture (Figure 6-5).

Beng Quan: 弸拳

6. Turn your body slightly to your right and back to the front as you circle your right hand clockwise in front of your abdomen and make a fist, palm facing in. Then step forward with your left leg and do Right Hand Beng to the west as your right leg follows (Figure 6-6).

146

Figure 6-3

Figure 6-4

Figure 6-5

Figure 6-6

Figure 6-7   Figure 6-8

Step Back for Heng Quan (Tui Bu Heng Quan): 退步橫拳
7. Move the left leg back into sitting crossed legs stance and do a Left Hand Heng (Figure 6-7).

Step Forward for Beng Quan (Shang Bu Beng Quan): 上步弸拳
8. Turn your body forward and readjust your front leg, and then step your right leg forward with Right Hand Beng to the west. While you are punching, the left leg follows and stamps to bounce the Jin upward to support the strike, and the left hand moves to the waist (Figure 6-8).

White Crane Spreads Its Wings (Bai He Liang Chi): 白鶴亮翅
9. Shift your weight to your left leg, move your right hand down over your left hand, both palms open and facing down (Figure 6-9).
10. Both hands rise together to face level, then open outward as you shift your weight forward (Figure 6-10).

Embrace the Moon on the Chest (Huai Zhong Bao Yue): 懷中抱月
11. Shift your weight back, bring both hands back to the abdomen, and strike the back of the right fist into the left palm as you stamp your right foot down just forward of your left foot (Figure 6-11).

Step Forward for Pao Quan (Jin Bu Pao Quan): 進步炮拳
12. Step 45 degrees to the right and do Left Hand Pao to the west (Figure 6-12).

Figure 6-9

Figure 6-10

Figure 6-11

Figure 6-12

Figure 6-13

Figure 6-14

Step Back for Zuan Quan (Tui Bu Zuan Quan): 退步鑽拳

13. Move your right foot back behind your left foot, pull the left fist to your abdomen, while circling your right forearm (elbow leading, palm of fist facing you) inward and then downward to block in front of your chest (Figure 6-13).

14. Pull your right fist to your abdomen as your left hand blocks down with an open palm. As you do this, your weight shifts back a little more and only the toe of the left foot is touching the ground (Figure 6-14).

15. The left hand continues to sink while the right drills upward and forward (Figure 6-15).

Step Forward for Pi Quan (Jin Bu Pi Quan): 進步劈拳

16. Step the left leg forward with the right leg following and at the same time execute Left Hand Pi Quan to the west (Figure 6-16).

Chicken Shape with Four Grabbings (Ji Xing Si Ba): 雞形四把

17. Step your left leg forward with the right leg following with a large step to just behind and to the side of the left leg. Only toes of the right foot touch the ground, and there is no weight on it. While stepping, move your left hand down to your abdomen and at the same time move your right hand underneath the left hand and push forward with the palm (Figure 6-17).

18. Step the right leg back (Figure 6-18).

Figure 6-15

Figure 6-16

Figure 6-17

Figure 6-18

Figure 6-19

Figure 6-20

19. Move the left foot back close to the right foot, touch the ground with the toes but keep all the weight on the right foot. While you are stepping, lower your right hand down to the abdomen and at the same time move your left hand underneath your right hand and push the palm forward (Figure 6-19).

20. Keeping your hands where they are in relation to your body, step your left leg 45 degrees to the left (southwest) (Figure 6-20).

21. Step your right leg up to the left leg with only the toes touching the ground and no weight on it. Lower your left hand down to the abdomen, and move your right hand underneath the left hand and push forward with the palm to the west (Figure 6-21).

22. Step your right foot 90 degrees to the right (northwest) (Figure 6-22).

Figure 6-21

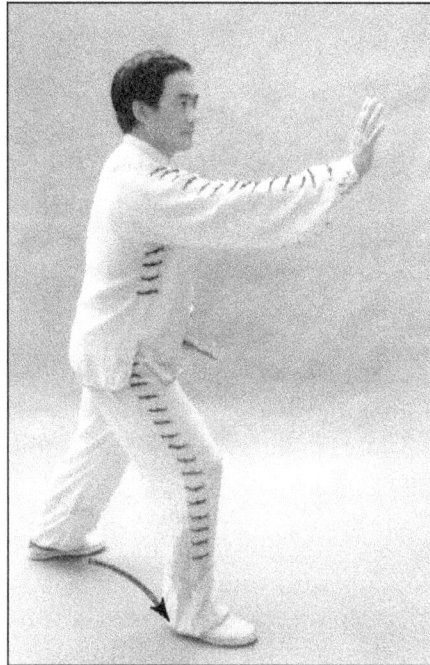

Figure 6-22

23. Step your left leg to join the right leg with the toes touching the ground and no weight on it. While you are stepping, lower your right hand down to your abdomen and at the same time move your left hand underneath your right hand and push your palm forward to the west (Figure 6-23).

Figure 6-23

Figure 6-24

Figure 6-25

Figure 6-26

Application: You are the one wearing the white uniform and facing your opponent with your left hand forward (Figure 6-24). When your opponent punches with his right fist, cover it downward with your left hand (Figure 6-25) and step your left leg forward while the right leg follows. While you are stepping, use your right hand to attack the opponent's face with a claw or grab (Figure 6-26).

Timing: The initial forward and back motions (Figures 6-17 to 6-19) are done slowly and deliberately, while the subsequent two moves to the corners are done quickly as one move.

Golden Rooster Steps Forward (Jin Ji Shang Bu): 金雞上步

24. Keeping your hands in front of your body, turn your body so that you are facing west, then step your left leg to the west (Figure 6-27).

25. Again do not move your hands, step forward with your right leg (Figure 6-28).

Golden Rooster Stands on One Leg (Jin Ji Du Li Shi): 金雞獨立式

26. Bring the left leg forward to touch the right leg half way up the calf (Figure 6-29).

Timing: After turning your body in #24 above, the two steps and are done quickly Pause for an instant with your leg up.

Golden Rooster Eats the Rice (Jin Ji Shi Mi): 金雞食米

27. Step your left leg forward (Figure 6-30).

Figure 6-27

Figure 6-28

Figure 6-29

Figure 6-30

Figure 6-31

Figure 6-32

28. Turn your body slightly to the right and back to the front as your right hand makes a circular motion and closes into a fist, palm facing in. Bring your right foot up to the side of the left foot and stamp as you punch forward with Jin, using the second knuckle of your middle finger. The left hand moves to the abdomen (Figure 6-31).

Golden Rooster Shakes its Scales (i.e., feathers)(Jin Ji Dou Lin): 金雞抖鱗

29. Open your right hand and make a clockwise-circling grabbing motion as if you were neutralizing and grabbing the opponent's punch, and at the same time raise your left hand to below the fight elbow (Figure 6-32).

Figure 6-33

Figure 6-34

Figure 6-35

30. Take a big step to the east with your right foot. As you shift your weight to it, pull your right elbow back to the east with the hand remaining at elbow height, and strike out to the west with your left palm (Figure 6-33).

Application: When your opponent punches with his right hand, intercept it and grab his right wrist (Figure 6-34). Then squat down and lock his left knee with your left hand (Figure 6-35). Finally, pull your right hand to your right and press your left hand to your left to make the opponent lose his balance and fall (Figure 6-36).

Figure 6-36

Figure 6-37

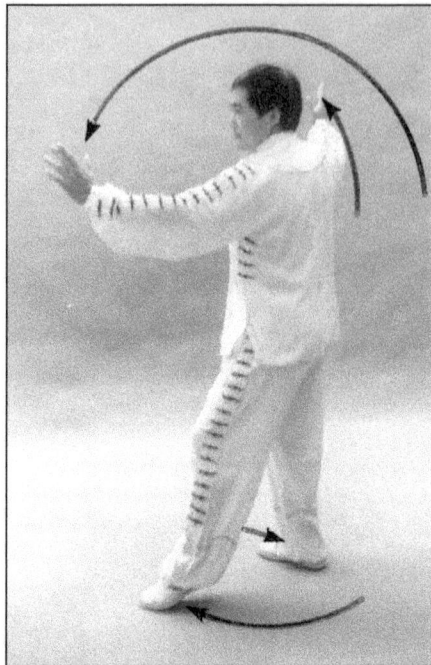

Figure 6-38

Golden Rooster on the Perch (Jin Ji Shang Jia): 金雞上架

31. Shift your weight to the left leg and pull your right leg back with toes touching the ground and facing the east. While you are doing this, swing your right hand down in front of you, back, and up. Then step the right leg forward again to the east as the fight hand continues to circle forward and down (Figure 6-37).

32. Pivot your fight foot on the heel, step your left leg forward as the left arm circles up, forward, and down, and the right arm circles down and to the rear (Figure 6-38).

33. Without interrupting the flow, pivot your left foot on the heel and step your fight leg forward to the side and slightly in front of the left leg, with only the toes touching the ground. At the same time, the right arm continues to circle over and down in front of the body, stopping in front of the groin, while the left hand moves to the front of the chest. Your body is facing north while your head is facing east, and all of your weight is on your left leg (Figure 6-39).

Application: When your opponent attacks with his right punch, swing your right arm from your left to your right to block the punch (Figure 6-40). If he steps back and throws a left hand punch, step forward with your left foot and, as you turn your body with the step, swing your left arm to block his attack (Figure 6-41). Seal his left arm downward with your left hand as you step forward with your right leg and strike downward with your right hand (Figure 6-42).

Figure 6-39

Figure 6-40

Figure 6-41

Figure 6-42

Figure 6-43

Figure 6-44

Figure 6-45

Golden Rooster Crows at Dawn (Jin Ji Bao Xiao): 金雞報曉

34. Step the right leg forward to the east and strike forward with the index finger edge of your right hand and pull your left hand down to your abdomen (Figure 6-43).

Application: Continuing from the last application, drop your right hand down and strike forward to the opponent's groin (Figure 6-44).

Tiger Shape Steps Forward Posture (Hu Xing Jin Bu Shi): 虎形進步式

35. Step the left foot to the northeast, bring your right leg in, and circle the hands together clockwise to the front of your face. You are now facing southeast (Figure 6-45).

36. Pull your right leg back toward the left leg and touch the toes to the ground. While doing this your hands continue to circle down to your Dan Tian. This reminds you to use the Qi from your Dan Tian (Figure 6-46).

Figure 6-46

Figure 6-47

Figure 6-48

Figure 6-49

37. Step the right leg forward to the southeast and at the same time push both hands forward. Your hands reach their position just as your foot strikes the ground (Figure 6-47).

Application: When your opponent attacks with his right hand (Figure 6-48), intercept it and guide it to your right with both hands (Figure 6-49), then step in and strike him with one or both hands in the side (Figure 6-50). Remember that your stepping is determined by the circumstances, and is not limited to what is practiced in the sequence.

Figure 6-50

Figure 6-51

Tiger Shape Changes the Posture (Hu Xing Huan Shi): 虎形換式

38. Step the right leg forward a small step to the east, and move your left leg east and touch the toes to the floor with the toes pointing northeast. At the same time turn your body to your left to face the northeast. Your hands rise and sink slightly so that as you turn they move in an arc (Figure 6-51).

39. Draw your left foot in and touch the toes next to your right foot and simultaneously continue the motion of your hands down to your Dan Tian (Figure 6-52).

40. Step your left leg forward to the northeast and at the same time push both hands forward (Figure 6-53).

Turn the Body for Horse Shape (Hui Shen Ma Xing): 回身馬形

41. Shift your weight to your fight foot and move your left foot to the southeast. Your hands start to move to your fight (Figure 6-54).

42. Shift your weight to your left foot as you continue rotating your body to the right. Move your fight foot in next to your left foot. While you are rotating your body and repositioning your legs, both hands circle in and down. The hands have closed into fists, and are palms down in front of your chest (Figure 6-55).

Figure 6-52

Figure 6-53

Figure 6-54

Figure 6-55

Figure 6-56

Figure 6-57

Figure 6-58

43. Step your fight leg to the northwest and strike out with fists and forearms (Figure 6-56).

Application: When your opponent attacks with a left sidekick, block it with both hands (Figure 6-57). Immediately step in with your right leg (the left leg follows) and strike or push the opponent's chest with both forearms (Figure 6-58).

Figure 6-59

Figure 6-60

Horse Shape Changes the Posture (Ma Xing Huan Shi): 馬形換式

44. Take a small step forward with your right leg, and start to turn your body to the left. The hands open and start to circle to the left (Figure 6-59).

45. Continue your turning, bring your left foot in next to the fight foot with the toes touching the ground. While you are repositioning your body and feet, both hands close into fists in front of your body (Figure 6-60).

46. Step your left foot to the southwest and strike out with fists and arms (Figure 6-61).

Figure 6-61

Figure 6-62

Figure 6-63

Beginning Posture of Bear Shape (Xiong Xing Qi Shi): 熊形起式

47. Move your fight fist down to your abdomen (Figure 6-62).

48. Step forward with the left leg and at the same time move your left hand down to your abdomen and move your right fist over the left hand and drill upward (Figure 6-63).

Figure 6-64

Application: When your opponent attacks you with his right punch, simply deflect the punch downward with your left hand while you punch to his chin with your right fist (Figure 6-64).

Eagle Shape Swoops Down (Ying Xing Luo Shi): 鷹形落式

49. Raise your right foot to half way up the left calf. At the same time, open your left hand and raise it inside the right arm until it reaches face height (Figure 6-65).

Figure 6-65

Figure 6-66

50. Open your right hand and turn the palm outward in a grabbing motion. Step your right leg to the northwest and pull your right hand down to your waist as your left hand presses down to knee level (Left Hand Pi). Your left hand is roughly an equal distance from both feet (Figure 6-66).

Figure 6-67

Application: When your opponent punches you with his right fist, use your right hand to intercept it and grab his right wrist. Pull his right hand to your right and at the same time use your left hand to lock his right shoulder and place your left leg in front of his right leg. Finally, step to your right with your right leg, and at the same time press your left hand down while pulling his right wrist to your right rear (Figure 6-67).

Figure 6-68   Figure 6-69

Beginning Posture of Bear Shape (Xiong Xing Qi Shi): 熊形起式

51. Step your right leg a small step forward as your left hand closes into a fist and starts to move upward (Figure 6-68).

52. Your left hand continues to drill upward (Figure 6-69).

Eagle Shape Swoops Down (Ying Xing Luo Shi): 鷹形落式

53. Raise your left foot to half way up the right calf. At the same time, open your right hand and raise it inside the left arm until it reaches face height (Figure 6-70).

54. Open your left hand and turn the palm outward in a grabbing motion. Step your left leg to the southwest and pull your left hand down to your waist as your right hand presses down to knee level (Right Hand Pi). Your right hand is roughly an equal distance from both feet (Figure 6-71).

Wildcat Climbs the Tree Backward (Li Mao Dao Shang Shu): 狸貓倒上樹

55. Shift your weight to your right foot and step to the north with your left foot. As your body turns to face the east, your right foot pivots and starts to pull back while your hands rise and sweep across the front of your body (Figure 6-72).

56. Bring your left hand down while your right hand closes into a fist and circles in and then drills out (Right Hand Zuan). At the same time, raise your right foot and kick forward with a drilling motion (Figure 6-73).

Figure 6-70

Figure 6-71

Figure 6-72

Figure 6-73

57. Step your right leg down into the sitting on crossed legs stance, and at the same time pull your right hand back and do left hand Pi (Figure 6-74).

Application: When your opponent attacks with his right fist, push his attack to your right with your left hand and at the same time punch him with your right fist and drill your right leg forward to kick his groin or knee (Figure 6-75). You can then attack his chest with your left hand Pi.

Right Beng Quan (You Beng Quan): 右弸拳

58. Your left leg steps forward and your right leg follows while pulling your left fist back to your abdomen and punch with your right fist (Figure 6-76).

Step Back for Heng Quan (Tui Bu Heng Quan): 退步横拳

59. Step your right leg back a small step (Figure 6-77).

60. Step your left leg back to form the sitting with crossed legs stance and at the same time pull your right fist back to your abdomen and strike with Left Hand Heng (Figure 6-78).

Black Tiger Exits From Cave (Hei Hu Chu Dong): 黑虎出洞

Figure 6-74

Figure 6-75

61. Turn your body to the left, step your right leg forward and follow with the left leg, and at the same time punch forward to the east with a right hand Beng while your left hand pulls back to your waist (Figure 6-79).

Figure 6-76

Figure 6-77

Figure 6-78

Figure 6-79

Figure 6-80

Figure 6-81

White Crane Spreads Its Wings (Bai He Liang Chi): 白鶴亮翅

62. Shift your weight back slightly to your left leg, and circle both hands down so that they cross at your waist with the right hand on the outside (Figure 6-80).

63. Shift your weight forward as the arms continue to circle up and out (Figure 6-81).

64. Shift your weight back. Continue to circle your left hand back to your waist as you pull your right hand in above your left hand. The back of the right fist hits the left palm as your right foot pulls in next to the left foot and stamps (Figure 6-82).

Figure 6-82

Figure 6-83

Step Forward for Pao Quan (Jin Bu Pao Quan): 進步炮拳

65. Step your right leg forward while the arms do Left Hand Pao. When you punch, stamp the left foot to bounce the Jin upward to the punching fist (Figure 6-83).

Wild Cat Climbs the Tree (Li Mo Shang Shu): 狸貓上樹

66. Shift all your weight to your left foot. Bring the right foot back and kick forward while dropping the left hand and drilling the right hand out in Zuan (Figure 6-84).

Figure 6-84

Figure 6-85

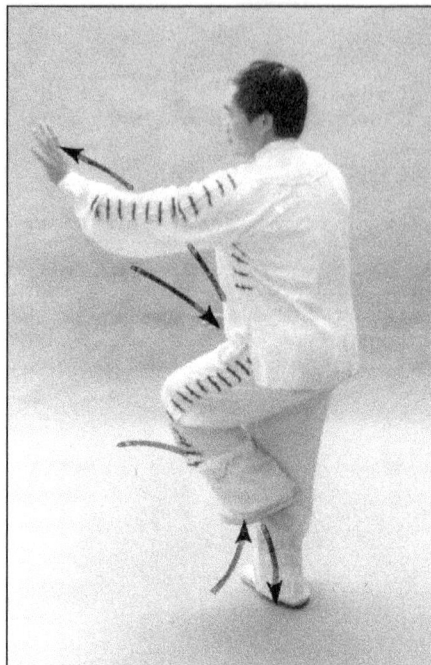

Figure 6-86

Golden Rooster Stands by One Leg (Jin Ji Du Li Shi): 金雞獨立式

67. While pulling back your kicking leg, also pull your right hand back and extend your left hand (Figure 6-85).

68. Drop your right foot to the ground and at the same time lift your left leg. As your fight foot hits the floor your Left Hand Pi reaches its position (Figure 6-86).

Gathering the Feet and Emitting the Palms (Bing Bu Chu Zhang): 并步出掌

69. Step your left leg forward and follow with the right. At the same time raise your left hand and then your fight hand over your head so that the back of the right hand hits the left palm (Figure 6-87).

Application: When your opponent attacks with his right hand, simply block upward with your left hand while stepping forward with your left leg and striking his groin with your right hand (Figure 6-88).

Figure 6-87

Figure 6-89

Figure 6-88

Figure 6-90

Step Back to Rein in the Horse (Tui Bu Le Ma Shi): 退步勒馬式

70. Step back with your right leg as your hands change into fists with the palms facing upward and start to draw in (Figure 6-89).

71. Pull your left leg back parallel to the right and bring both fists palm up to the front of your abdomen (Figure 6-90).

Figure 6-91

Figure 6-92

Application: Continuing from the last form, you can grab the opponent's hair and pull down while stepping back (Figure 6-91).

Tiger Shape Steps Forward (Hu Xing Jin Bu): 虎形進步

72. Step your right leg forward and push forward with both palms (Figure 6-92).

Figure 6-93

Application: Continuing from the last application, if your opponent resists and pulls his head backward, simply let go of his hair, follow his backward motion, step forward and push or strike his chest with both hands (Figure 6-93).

Timing: #70 is done slowly and deliberately, #71 is done quickly and firmly to draw Qi into your Dan Tian, and #72 is done quickly and with force.

Step Forward Pao Quan (Jin Bu Pao Quan): 進步炮拳

73. Take a small step forward with your right leg, then draw your left foot forward to the side of the right foot, with the toes touching the ground, and at the same time bring your hands in to your waist. Then step your left leg to your left front and let your right leg follow and do Right Hand Pao to the northeast (Figure 6-94).

Figure 6-94

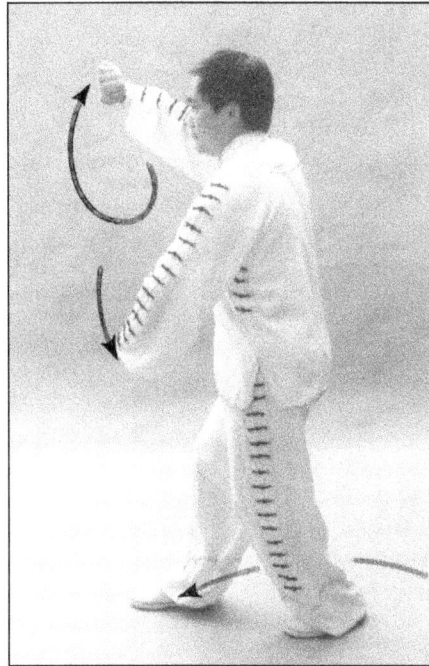

Figure 6-95

Dragon and Tiger Mutually Intersect (Long Hu Xiang Jiao): 龍虎相交

74. Step your right leg to the east and swing your right arm in a circular block to your right as your left arm circles down to your waist (Figure 6-95).

75. Step your left leg forward and swing your left arm past your face in a counterclockwise, circular block, and at the same time let your right arm continue downward until the fist is at the waist (Figure 6-96).

Figure 6-96

Figure 6-97

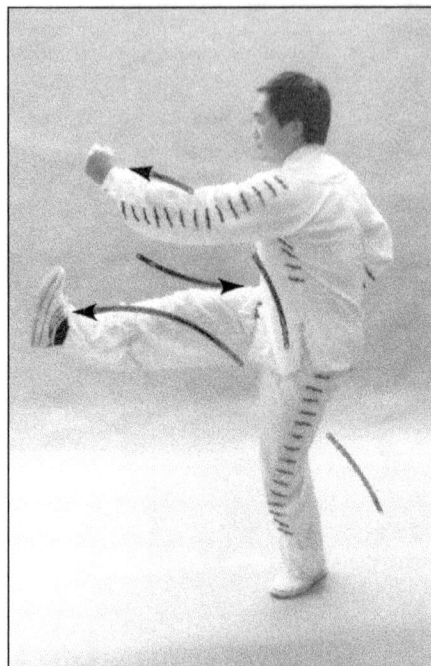

Figure 6-98

76. As your weight settles into your left leg, the motion of the arms continues smoothly into Right Hand Beng. The left fist moves to the waist (Figure 6-97).

77. Kick the right leg out and at the same time punch forward with the left hand and draw the right hand to the waist (Figure 6-98).

78. Drop the fight leg to the ground and at the same time pull the left fist to the abdomen and punch forward to the east with the fight hand (Figure 6-99).

Figure 6-99

Figure 6-100

Figure 6-101

White Crane Spreads Its Wings (Bai He Liang Chi): 白鶴亮翅

79. As you shift your weight to the rear foot, move both hands to the waist, fight hand on the outside (Figure 6-100).

80. Shift your weight to the front foot as you spread both hands up and to the sides (Figure 6-101).

Embrace the Moon in the Chest (Huai Zhong Bao Yue): 懷中抱月

81. Shift your weight back. Continue to circle your left hand back to your waist as you pull your right hand in above your left hand. The back of the fight fist hits the left palm as your fight foot pulls in next to the left foot and stamps (Figure 6-102).

Figure 6-102

179

Figure 6-103

Figure 6-104

Sparrow Hawk Enters the Woods (Yao Zi Ru Lin): 鷂子入林

82. This movement is also called "Jump and Exchange Legs for Pao Quan." Jump up and twist your body to the fight, switching your legs simultaneously so that left leg is in front while the fight leg is in back. As you are doing this, block up with the right arm and punch out with the left arm for Pao (Figure 6-103).

Sparrow Hawk Flies into the Sky (Yao Zi Zuan Tian): 鷂子鑽天

83. Step forward with the right leg. Your right hand moves down to your waist and strikes forward with the middle knuckle of the index finger for Right Hand Zuan. The left fist drops slightly to below the right elbow, palm facing down (Figure 6-104).

Figure 6-105

Figure 6-106

Sparrow Hawk Turns Its Body (Yao Zi Fan Shen): 鷂子翻身

84. Turn your body 180 degrees to the rear (west) and circle your right hand over your head (Figure 6-105).

85. The right hand continues and blocks down while the left hand drills up and forward with Zuan. The feet pivot as needed. The right hand ends up under the left elbow (Figure 6-106).

Figure 6-107

Figure 6-108

Figure 6-109

Figure 6-110

Swallow Enters the Wood (Yan Zi Chuan Lin): 燕子穿林

86. As you start to turn your body to the rear, raise your right arm while pulling the left arm back (Figure 6-107).

87. Continue the motion by bringing your right arm down, the knuckle of the index finger still protruding, while the left hand moves to your abdomen. The right fist is palm upward (Figure 6-108).

Application: You have punched at your opponent with your right hand and he has intercepted it and is pulling it down (Figure 6-109). Simply shift your body forward, lift up your right arm and circle it around his neck and lock it. Then drop to your right knee to take him down (Figure 6-110).

Figure 6-111

Figure 6-112

Figure 6-113

Figure 6-114

Swallow Seizes the Water (Yan Zi Chao Shui): 燕子抄水

88. Continue to circle the right fist to your right ear as you face back to the west (Figure 6-111).

89. Lower your body with the weight mostly on the right foot, and extend your left fist down along the length of your left leg. The knuckle of the index finger is protruding, and the palm is facing to your right. The right fist moves to the waist (Figure 6-112).

Application: When your opponent punches with his right fist, intercept it with your left forearm and right hand while stepping your left foot behind his right leg. Your right hand immediately grabs his wrist (Figure 6-113).

Immediately squat down on your right leg and pull his right arm down with you, and simultaneously place your left hand behind his left knee (Figure 6-114). Finally, stand up and push him to his rear with your body while pulling his left knee forward (Figure 6-115).

Figure 6-115

Sparrow Hawk Binds Its Body (Yao Zi Shu Shen): 鷂子束身

90. Step and stamp the right foot next to the left foot while lifting the left foot up, and at the same time the right fist strikes forward palm up (Figure 6-116).

91. Keeping your body in the same location, step the left leg forward and immediately slide the right leg backward. As you are doing this, raise your fight fist palm inward and punch forward with your left hand. The middle knuckles of both index fingers are protruding (Figure 6-117).

Figure 6-116

Application: When your opponent attacks with a fight punch, block it downward with your left hand (Figure 6-118). Immediately step and stamp your right leg forward and use your right hand to attack his groin (Figure 6-119). If he pulls his body back to avoid your attack and punches with his left, you can block it with your right hand and punch with your left hand.

Cat Washes Its Face (Mao Xi Lian): 貓洗臉

92. Step your left foot to the rear while brushing across your body with your open right hand. Your left hand opens and withdraws to your abdomen. All your weight is on your left foot, with only the toes of the right foot touching the floor (Figure 6-120).

93. Your right hand continues its motion and lowers to your abdomen, while your left hand brushes across your body (Figure 6-121).

Figure 6-117

Figure 6-118

Figure 6-119

Figure 6-120

Figure 6-121

Figure 6-122

Figure 6-123

Application: These movements are simply used for defense. When your opponent punches, you sit back and brush the punches away (Figures 6-122 and 6-123). All of your weight is on your rear leg so that the front leg can kick while you are blocking.

Black Tiger Exits the Cave (Hei Hu Chu Dong): 黑虎出洞

94. Step forward to the east with the right leg and punch out with the right fist while pulling the left fist back to the abdomen (Figure 6-124).

Application: Continuing from the last application, if you do not kick you may simply step forward and punch to his liver area (Figure 6-125).

Figure 6-124

Figure 6-125

Figure 6-126

Figure 6-127

Wind Blows the Lotus Leaf (Feng Bai He Ye): 風擺荷葉

95. Shift your weight to your rear and bring both open hands down in a circular motion (Figure 6-126).

96. Step your right leg across the front of your body to the southeast and move into a sitting on crossed legs stance. As you do this your hands circle to your left, up, and past your face to your right, until the right hand is in front of you at eye level and your left hand is near your right armpit (Figure 6-127).

Figure 6-128

Figure 6-129

Turn the Body for Pi Quan (Zhuan Shen Pi Quan): 轉身劈拳

97. As your weight shifts toward your right leg, the right hand circles over the head. You are now facing the east (Figure 6-128).

98. As your weight continues to shift to the right leg, the right hand blocks down in front of your face, and the left hand comes up inside it, palm facing you (Figure 6-129).

99. Finally, step the left leg forward for Left Hand Pi (Figure 6-130).

Sparrow Hawk Ascends into the Sky (Yao Zi Zuan Tian): 鷂子鑽天

100. Step forward with your right leg and raise your left leg as you lower your left arm and drill forward and upward with Right Hand Zuan (Figure 6-131).

Sparrow Hawk Turns Its Body (Yao Zi Fan Shen): 鷂子翻身

101. Turn your body 180 degrees to the west while your right arm circles over your head and starts to sink (Figure 6-132).

102. Step forward to the west with your left leg while the right hand continues to drop downward and the left fist drills upward and forward for Zuan (Figure 6-133).

Figure 6-130

Figure 6-131

Figure 6-132

Figure 6-133

Figure 6-134

Figure 6-135

Sparrow Hawk Holds the Seeds (Yao Zi Shu Zi): 鷂子束子

103. Bring your right leg forward to the side of the left leg, with the foot off the ground. Your right fist moves to your waist (Figure 6-134).

104. Stamp your right leg down and at the same time lift up your left leg. While you are doing this, pull your left fist to your waist and punch forward with your right fist, palm up (Figure 6-135).

105. Keeping your body in the same location, step your left leg forward while sliding your right leg to the rear. While doing this, block upward with your right fist and punch forward with your left hand (Figure 6-136).

Golden Rooster Shakes Its Wings (Jin Ji Dou Chi): 金雞抖翅

106. Turn to the north and start swinging your arms in a circular motion. The fight elbow swings to your upper rear, while the left arm swings down and forward. Turn your body and swing your arms in circles so that your elbows rise and then strike to your rear, while the other arm swings down and forward to balance the motion (Figures 6-137 to 6-139). Circle your arms slowly as you do three strikes, and then speed up and do three strikes with Jin.

Figure 6-136

Figure 6-137

Figure 6-138

Figure 6-139

Figure 6-140

Figure 6-141

Figure 6-142

Figure 6-143

Application: If you are being held from the rear in a bearhug, immediately expand your body and arms to the sides (Figure 6-140). Shake and rotate until both his arms are loose (Figures 6-141 and 6-142). Once your opponent has lost his hold, use your elbows and the body's turning power to strike or bounce him backward (Figure 6-143).

Figure 6-144

Figure 6-145

Close Both Legs to Conclude (Bing Bu Shou Shi): 并步收式

107. Step your right leg to the rear (Figure 6-144).

108. Move your left leg back next to the fight leg while raising both arms in a large circular motion. Your body faces northeast (Figure 6-145).

109. Both hands move up and down, and close into fists as they pass your chest and end at your abdomen. While your hands are lowering, turn your body and right toes to face the north. Stand still with your mind quiet for a few seconds (Figure 6-146).

Figure 6-146

CHAPTER 7
An Shen Pao 安身炮

7.1 INTRODUCTION

Traditionally, in order to train a student to be a proficient martial artist, certain training procedures are followed. Normally in the beginning stage a student will receive from six months to one year of the most basic training, such as fundamental stances and stepping. This builds up the strength of the legs, the root, and the basic postural requirements for further physical training. In addition, the student also learns to build up his patience, perseverance, and endurance.

Once he has completed the fundamental training both physically and mentally, he will then start to learn sequences or routines. These contain the essence of the art, and they are the means by which the art is preserved through the generations. Sequences and routines enable the student to master the techniques, and to become familiar with the fighting strategy and movements of the style. They also let the student train speed and the Jins, and develop a sense of enemy.

When a student has reached a high level of understanding through the training of sequences, he will then start to learn how to apply the techniques in a fight. Before the actual sparring training, however, he will usually learn prearranged fighting sets. These are designed to give the student a feel for real fighting situations. They teach him to keep a safe distance from the opponent, and how to execute timely and accurate techniques. Only after a student has practiced many fighting sets will he have built up the natural reactions which are necessary in a fight, and only then will he become involved in sparring without prearranged techniques.

An Shen Pao (安身炮)(Secure Body Strike) is a well-known Xingyiquan fighting set. It will help you to understand the strategy, principles, and theory of Xingyiquan fighting, and it will also familiarize you with how the techniques are set up. The final goal of the training is to build up correct natural reactions. In order to reach this goal, you must practice with different people. This is because everyone has a different reach, speed, habits, and stride. If you are able to practice with different people until the forms are smooth and your reactions are natural, you will have surely built a firm foundation for sparring.

Remember that An Shen Pao offers only typical examples of Xingyiquan applications. You should not be restricted by its forms and applications. It teaches only

Figure 7-1

Figure 7-2

Figure 7-3

Figure 7-4

the essence of the art. Once you understand the essence of this fighting set, you will be able to open your own door and find your own particular field of study and practice. Only then will you eventually be able to become a real master.

7.2 AN SHEN PAO

1. Black and White stand facing opposite directions about three steps apart. Their feet form slightly slanted V's (Figure 7-1).

2. Both Black and White raise their hands slowly from the sides with palms facing upward (Figure 7-2).

3. The hands continue to circle up and around. As they approach chest height, they close into fists. Black and White continue to lower their hands until they reach the Lower Dan Tian, palms down, then they turn their heads and look at each other (Figure 7-3).

4. Black and White twist their bodies to face each other, and as they turn they raise their right fists to chin height, drilling the palms upward (Figure 7-4).

Figure 7-5

Figure 7-6

Figure 7-7

Figure 7-8

5. Black and White raise their left fists palm upward, and then push the open palms out along the right arm and step forward into the Three Body Posture (San Ti Shi)(Figure 7-5).

6. White steps his left leg forward and follows with the right leg, executing a Right Hand Beng to Black's solar plexus. His left hand moves back to his abdomen. When Black sees White's punch he takes a small step backward with his right leg and raises his left leg, and at the same time uses his left hand to brush White's punch to the side. As he deflects the punch he also withdraws his right hand to his waist (Figure 7-6).

7. Black then steps down with his left leg and uses his right hand to punch (Beng) White's solar plexus (Figure 7-7).

8. White immediately pulls his right hand back to grab Black's wrist and at the same time pushes his left hand forward (Pi) to Black's shoulder (Figure 7-8).

Figure 7-9

Figure 7-10

Figure 7-11

Figure 7-12

9. Black pull his right arm back to block White's Pi and at the same time uses his left hand to strike White's face (Figure 7-9).

10. White slides his right leg back and step to his right to avoid Black's strike while at the same time circling his left hand down and then up to intercept Black's attack (Figure 7-10).

11. White continues his movement and steps in with his right leg to Black's left side. His left hand directs Black's left hand down and his right hand pushes (Pi) Black's left shoulder (Figure 7-11).

12. Black pulls his left hand back to intercept White's Pi while pulling his left leg back (Figure 7-12).

13. Black pulls Whites right wrist down with his left hand, step in with his right leg, and does Right Hand Pi to White's Face (Figure 7-13).

14. White raises both hands and twists his arms and body to the left to intercept and block Black's attack. His left palm faces out and his right palm faces towards him (Figure 7-14).

15. Black pulls his right hand back and uses Left Hand Pi to strike White's face (Figure 7-15).

16. White twists his body to the right and block Black's attack with both fists. As he does this he rotates both arms so that his left palm faces him and his right palm faces out (Figure 7-16).

Figure 7-13

Figure 7-14

Figure 7-15

Figure 7-16

Figure 7-17

Figure 7-18

17. White continues his movement and drops his right fist under his left elbow to punch Black's abdomen, while his left hand is still blocking Black's left hand (Figure 7-17).

18. Black slides his left leg back slightly and raises his right leg while directing White's punch upward with his right hand at White's wrist and his left hand at the elbow (Figure 7-18).

Figure 7-19

Figure 7-20

Figure 7-21

Figure 7-22

19. Black steps down with his right leg and does Right Hand Beng to White's solar plexus (Figure 7-19).

20. White shifts his weight back, pulls his right hand back, circles it clockwise up and grabs Black's right wrist. At the same time he raises his right leg, and uses his left hand to push Black's shoulder down (Figure 7-20).

21. White continues the movement, steps his right leg down, slides his left hand down to Black's right wrist, and strikes at Black's chest with his right palm (Figure 7-21).

22. Black steps his right leg back into the sitting on crossed legs stance, pulls his right hand back, and drills it upward to intercept White's attack (Figure 7-22).

23. White continues his attack by stepping his left leg forward and following with his right leg. While he is stepping, he raises his left hand from under his right elbow and pushes Black's right arm up and to the side, and uses his right fist to punch (Pao) Black's chest (Figure 7-23).

24. Black immediately adjusts the distance by shifting his weight to his right leg and leaving only his left toes touching the ground. While shifting his weight he also turns his body and intercepts White's right hand with his left hand. His right fist pulls back to his Lower Dan Tian (Figure 7-24).

Figure 7-23

Figure 7-24

Figure 7-25

Figure 7-26

Figure 7-27

Figure 7-28

25. White drops his left hand to deflect Black's left wrist to the side, and steps forward with his right leg while circling his right hand to chop to the left side of Black's neck or face (Figure 7-25).

26. Black pulls his left hand up and intercepts White's attack (Figure 7-26).

27. White uses his left hand to push Black's block to the side (Figure 7-27).

28. While pushing Black's left hand outward, White moves his right hand under Black's arm and strikes at Black's face with his right palm. He also takes a small step forward with his right foot to get into striking range (Figure 7-28).

Figure 7-29

Figure 7-30

Figure 7-31

Figure 7-32

29. Black pulls his left hand back while pushing White's attack to the left with his right hand (Figure 7-29).

30. Black continues the movement and raises his left hand inside his own right hand to grab White's wrist or push it to the side (Figure 7-30).

31. Black then steps his right leg in and adjust his left leg while using the back of his right hand to strike White's face (Figure 7-31).

32. White steps his right leg back, pulls his right hand back and drills it up to intercept Black's attack (Figure 7-32).

33. White continues his movement, grabs and pulls Black's right arm down as he turns to his right, and takes a small step forward as he strikes Black's face with his left hand (Figure 7-33).

34. Black shifts his weight back to his left leg and circles his right hand to intercept White's attack (Figure 7-34).

35. Black continues his movement by raising his right leg. While his right hand is directing White's left arm down, his left hand pushes forward and down to White's shoulder (Figure 7-35).

36. Black continues his movement by stepping his right leg down and striking White's face with his right hand (Figure 7-36).

Figure 7-33

Figure 7-34

Figure 7-35

Figure 7-36

Figure 7-37

Figure 7-38

37. White slides his right leg back slightly and follows with the left leg to avoid Black's attack, while pulling his left arm back and drilling it up to intercept Black's attack (Figure 7-37).

38. White then steps in with his right leg, his left hand pushes Black's right arm up, and at the same time he strikes Black's groin with the forward edge of his right hand (Figure 7-38).

Figure 7-39

Figure 7-40

Figure 7-41

Figure 7-42

39. Black steps his right leg back, pulls his right hand down to grab White's right wrist, and pushes his left hand forward and downward to White's right shoulder as he steps in with his left foot to the outside of White's right foot (Figure 7-39).

40. White pulls his right hand back and directs Black's push upward, and at the same time strikes Black's face his left hand (Figure 7-40).

41. Black raises his right hand to intercept White's attack (Figure 7-41).

42. White hooks Black's right hand to the side with his left hand and at the same time uses his right hand to strike Black's face (Figure 7-42).

43. Black immediately pulls his right hand back to intercept White's attack while bringing his left hand to his abdomen (Figure 7-43).

44. Black then strikes White's face with his left palm (Figure 7-44).

45. White shifts his weight back, pulls his right hand back and uses it to grab Black's left wrist and pull it down (Figure 7-45).

Figure 7-43

Figure 7-44

Figure 7-45

Figure 7-46

Figure 7-47

Figure 7-48

46. White continues his movement by raising his right leg and pushing his left hand forward to Black's shoulder (Figure 7-46).

47. White continues, stepping his right leg down while using his right hand to strike Black's face (Figure 7-47).

48. Black steps his left leg back into the sitting on crossed legs stance while drilling his right hand upward to intercept White's attack (Figure 7-48).

Figure 7-49

Figure 7-50

Figure 7-51

Figure 7-52

49. White steps his left leg forward while lifting his left hand upward to push Black's arm up and to the side (Figure 7-49).

50. White continues his movement by circling his left arm down and squeezing Black's right arm under his armpit while using his right palm to attack the left side of Black's face (Figure 7-50).

51. Black turns his body to his left and shifts his weight to his left leg, while at the same time intercepting White's strike with both arms. His left palm faces out, and his right palm faces in (Figure 7-51).

52. White pulls his right hand back and attacks the right side of Black's face with his left palm. Black twists his body to his right and blocks White's strike with both hands (the reverse of Figure 7-51)(Figure 7-52).

53. Black continues the previous movement, and uses his right hand to punch Black's solar plexus (Figure 7-53).

54. White steps his right leg back slightly and follows with his left leg, touching the toes only to the floor, and directs Black's punch downward with his left hand (Figure 7-54).

55. White steps his left leg forward and uses his right hand to push Black's right hand down and to his left (Figure 7-55).

Figure 7-53

Figure 7-54

Figure 7-55

Figure 7-56

Figure 7-57

Figure 7-58

56. White hops forward with his left leg and kicks to Black's abdomen with his right foot. As he is doing this he attacks Black's face with his left and then right hands in a continuous, circular motion (Figure 7-56).

57. Black retreats with three steps, moving each time into the sitting on crossed legs stance, and blocks White's right hand by drilling his right hand up (Figure 7-57).

58. Right after White's right leg steps down, he immediately steps his left leg in and blocks Black's right arm up with his left hand, and gets ready to strike with Pao (Figure 7-58).

Figure 7-59

Figure 7-60

Figure 7-61

Figure 7-62

59. White continues the movement by attacking Black's solar plexus with a Right Hand Pao (Figure 7-59).

60. Black turns his body to his right and at the same time blocks White's punch downward with his left hand (Figure 7-60).

61. White drops his left hand down to cover Black's left hand, and at the same time attacks the left side of Black's face with his right palm (Figure 7-61).

62. Black raises his left hand and stops White's strike by grabbing and pushing White's right shoulder (Figure 7-62).

63. White steps his left leg back and moves his right leg in slightly while circling his right hand up to free his shoulder from Black's grab (Figure 7-63).

64. White continues his movement by lifting his right leg up while grabbing Black's left wrist and pulling it down with his right hand and pushing forward and down to Black's left shoulder with his left hand (Figure 7-64).

65. White then steps his right leg down and at the same time strikes Black's face with his right hand (Figure 7-65).

Figure 7-63

Figure 7-64

Figure 7-65

Figure 7-66

Figure 7-67

Figure 7-68

66. Black shifts his weight back and circles his left hand up to intercept White's strike (Figure 7-66).

67. Black slides his left leg forward and uses his right hand to strike the left side of White's face (Figure 7-67).

68. White turns his body to the left and blocks Black's strike with both hands (Figure 7-68).

Figure 7-69

Figure 7-70

Figure 7-71

Figure 7-72

69. Black then pulls his right hand back and at the same time swings his left hand to attack the right side of White's face (Figure 7-69).

70. White turns his body to his right and blocks Black's attack with both hands (Figure 7-70).

71. Immediately after blocking, White uses his right hand to Beng Black's solar plexus while pulling his left hand back to his abdomen (Figure 7-71).

72. Black steps his right leg back slightly and follows with the left leg, and circles his right hand to cover White's punch (Figure 7-72).

73. Black continues the movement by pushing his left palm forward and downward toward White's right shoulder (Figure 7-73).

74. Black then steps his left leg forward as his left hand slides down White's right arm, and follows with his right leg, while at the same time uses his right hand to Beng White's solar plexus (Figure 7-74).

Figure 7-73

Figure 7-74

Figure 7-75

75. White steps his right leg back and lifts his left leg while using his left hand to direct Black's attack to the side (Figure 7-75).

If you wish, you can continue the sequence. White can now attack as Black did in Figure 7-6, and Black can follow with the moves that White used. You can repeat the sequence as often as you wish, switching sides each time. When you wish to stop:

Ending: To end the exchanges from Figure 7-74: Black slides his right leg back, then pulls his left leg back to it so that he ends facing the same direction as in the beginning. He then turns his palms up, raises them over his head, turns the palms down and lowers them. The hands change to fists as they pass the chest, and continue down to the Dan Tian. White steps his right leg back, and pulls his left leg back to it. He is now facing the same direction as in the beginning. He then raises and lowers his arms as Black did.

Conclusion 結論

We have tried to introduce the essence of Xingyiquan to you through translations of the documents that are available to us. Because of the profound nature of these documents, we have only been able to offer a superficial level of commentary on them. We deeply believe that if you practice conscientiously, over the years you will accumulate enough knowledge and experience to take you beyond the level of our commentary. These poems and songs retain the essence and the root of the entire Xingyiquan system. If you have taken yourself away from these theories and principles, the style you practice can no longer be called Xingyiquan.

We would like to remind you again that the sequences and the fighting set introduced in this book are only meant to introduce you to the correct concepts. There are many other sequences available from books and experienced masters. We believe that as long as you remain humble, and study and ponder carefully, you can become a real Xingyiquan master.

It is recommended that if you have read through the main text of this book, you should start to read and study Yue, Fei's *Ten Important Theses*. They will lead you to a deeper level of understanding during the course of your practice.

Yue, Fei's Ten Important Theses 岳武穆形意拳十要論

In this Appendix we would like to introduce Marshal Yue, Fei's Ten Important Theses on Xingyiquan. These ten theses can be considered the essence or the root of the art. We can clearly see that all of the available documents and books written in the last 60 years derive almost all of their theories and principles from these theses.

Like other ancient documents which have been passed down to us, they are very difficult to translate and even harder to write commentary for. We would like to point out a few things. First, many subjects are repeated several times in different theses. Since this document has been passed down through a period of over eight hundred years, these repetitions may have occurred during the process of copying, or they may stem from revisions by past masters. Second, there are several places in the text that are not clearly expressed. These may be due to copyists' mistakes or mistakes that cropped up during the years of being passed down orally. Most of the people in ancient times could not read, so the secrets had to be passed down orally and memorized. Third, because of our limited background and knowledge, the commentary may not always explain the text adequately. Also, many sections are open to several explanations, and another experienced master may offer other ideas. Fourth, it is very difficult to find good English translations for many Chinese words, especially those which describe or explain spiritual feelings. We will try to explain these in the commentary by using examples. We hope that this will lead you to a feeling for what the words actually mean.

Yue, Fei's theses include:

1. Thesis of Integrity (Yi Tong Lun) 一統論
2. Thesis of Yin and Yang (Yin Yang Lun) 陰陽論
3. Thesis of the Three Sections (San Jie Lun) 三節論
4. Thesis of the Four Extremities (Si Shao Lun) 四梢論
5. Thesis of the Five Phases (Wu Xing Lun) 五形論
6. Thesis of the Six Combinations (Liu He Lun) 六合論
7. Thesis of the Seven Advancings (Qi Jin Lun) 七進論

8. Thesis of the Body's Maneuvers (Shen Fa Lun) 身法論

9. Thesis of Stepping (Bu Fa Lun) 步法論

10. Thesis of Fighting (Jiao Shou Lun) 交手論

1. Thesis of Integrity (Yi Tong Lun) 一‧一統論

From the beginning, (all that is) discrete must have its unification, the divided must be combined. Therefore, between heaven and earth, all that is disordered has its abode, all the thousand branches and the confusion of ten thousand endings, all have their origin. This is because one root divides into ten thousand branches, and ten thousand branches all belong to one root. (All of these) events are the natural (way).

從來散之必有其統也，分之必有其合也。以故天壤間四
面八方，紛紛者各有其屬，千頭萬緒，攘攘者自有其源。
蓋一本散為萬殊，而萬殊咸歸於一本，事有必然者。

It can be seen throughout the seven thousand years of Chinese history that the natural course of things is for that which is divided to finally be united, and that which is united to again be divided. However, no matter how many times things change or divide, they all originally came from one root.

This implies that although the events that happen in this world are sometimes random and confused and sometimes unified and clear, there are still only two tendencies: toward Yin and toward Yang. That which is already random (extreme Yang) must be gradually combined (toward Yin), and that which is already unified (extreme Yin) will again gradually be divided and become random. This Yin and Yang theory describes the way things naturally function in this universe. If you can really comprehend this theory, your mind will be clear and you will be able to adjust yourself to fit into this natural cycle.

(If) this theory is applied to the martial arts, it (i.e., the dividing) is also numerous. The important point is (that) the thousands of changes and the ten thousand variations (are) nothing but postures and nothing but Qi. Although the postures cannot be classified, the Qi however is one.

且武事之論，亦甚繁矣。而要之，千變萬化，無往非勢，
即無往非氣。勢雖不類，而氣歸一。

Although there are thousands of techniques ("postures") and variations in the martial arts, their root remains the same. You may divide these postures into Yin and Yang (i.e., attacking and defending, extending and withdrawing, etc.), however, there is only one root within this Yin and Yang, and it is nothing else but Qi. It is the Qi which makes and varies the Yin and Yang. Without this Qi, the Yin and Yang would lose their root. In the martial arts, all of the numerous techniques are nothing but variations of postures and how you move, and all of these come down to how you move your Qi.

About what "one" means, from (your) top to the bottom of the feet, internally there are viscera, bowels, tendons, and bones. Externally, there are muscles, skin, the five sensing organs, and hundreds of skeletons (i.e., bones), mutually combined and become one. When struck will not open, when hit will not decompose. (When) the top wishes to move, the bottom automatically follows. The bottom wishes to move, the top will automatically lead. (When) the top and the bottom move, the center section will attack. (When) the center section moves, the top and the bottom will coordinate. Internal and external are combined, the front and the rear mutually required. This is what is called "threading into one."

夫所謂一者，從上至足底，內有臟腑筋骨，外有肌肉皮
膚五官百骸，相聯而為一貫者也。破之而不開，撞之而
不散。上欲動而下自隨之。下欲動而上自領之。上下動
而中節攻之。中節動而上下合之。內外相連，前後相需，
所謂一貫者，其斯之謂歟。

In Xingyiquan, the entire body from top to bottom, from front to rear, from inside to outside, is all combined together as one. This is achieved by connecting the Qi throughout the body ("threading into one"). Normally the Qi seems to be disconnected because the mind does not perceive it as being one. The top here means the head which includes the mind, the center section implies the hands and the waist, and the bottom section indicates the legs. When the Qis in the different parts of your body are threaded into one, then when one place moves, the entire body will follow in coordination. You can see that in the martial arts the primary root of everything is the Qi.

This cannot be reached through force or done (simply) from imitating. When it is time to be calm, it is quiet and transparent. In this position, (you) are steady like a mountain. When it is time to move, like thunder and like (a mountain) collapsing. The speed of emitting (Jin) is like lighting. In addition, when calm, nothing is not calm. The surface and the internal, the top and the bottom, all without disorder and the meaning (i.e., the way) of inhibiting each other (i.e., stagnation). When moving, nothing does not move. The left and the right, the front and the rear, all without pulling (dragging), and the shape of swiftly moving around. It is just like water flowing downward, it is so powerful that nothing is able to stop it. It is like (a cannon is) fired internally, when (it is) shot, (you are) not fast enough to cover your ears. Without considering thinking, without bothering to plan, simply reach the goal without expectation. (When) this (goal) is reached without intention, then isn't it the natural way?

而要非勉強以致之，襲焉而為之也。當時而靜，寂然湛
然，居其所而穩如山岳。當時而動，如雷如塌，出乎爾
而疾如閃電。且靜無不靜，表裡上下，全無參差牽掛之
意。動無不動，左右前後，並無抽扯游移之形。洵乎若
水之就下，沛然而莫之能禦，若火之內攻，發之而不及
掩耳。不假思索，不煩擬議，誠不期然而然，莫之致而
至，是豈無所自而云然乎。

All of the above accomplishments cannot be achieved through force or imitation. You need to really comprehend the meaning of the theory and experience the actual feeling of the postures, then gradually every posture and movement will become natural and automatic. At this stage, when you are calm you are steady and rooted like a mountain, and when you move your power is like a collapsing mountain and you are as fast as lighting.

When you are calm, your entire body is calm from the inside (mind) to the surface (postures). Once you start to move, there is no stagnation and no confusion. You move as fast and smoothly as water rushing down a hillside, and as powerfully as a cannonball. All of this comes from your natural reactions. You do not have time to think or to anticipate. They are done without plan or expectation.

> *Because the Qi must be accumulated daily to gain benefit, Gong (i.e., Qigong) is trained for a long time (before) success. In contemplating the way one passes through the holy door, one must wait until one has listened repeatedly and gained sufficient knowledge and has reached the stage where he suddenly comprehends, and has not ignored achieving through thorough training, then he knows that these things are not (divided into) difficult and easy. The achievement can (only) be reached as an end by itself, (it) cannot be (done) through waiting and (it) cannot be speeded up. Follow the steps and catch the pace, advancing according to the (proper) order. Only then will the organs, skeletonbones, limbs, and joints connect automatically, and the top and bottom, the external and internal not have difficulty communicating. Then those randoms will be gathered and those divided will be unified. The four limbs and hundreds of skeletonbones will all belong to one Qi.*

> 蓋氣以日積而有益，功以久練而始成。觀聖門一貫之傳，
> 必俟多聞強識之後，豁然之境，不廢格物致知之功，是
> 知事無難易，功惟自盡，不可躐等，不可急遽，按步就
> 步，循次而進，夫而後官骸肢節，自有通貫，上下表裡，
> 不難聯絡。庶乎散者統之，分者合之，四體百骸，終歸
> 於一氣而已矣。

All of the training can not be done in one day. It takes years of training and accumulating experiences. Only then will you really comprehend the theory and understand the training. Finally, all of the training will become a natural part of you, and only then can all of the random and disconnected parts be threaded together by the one Qi.

---

2. Thesis of Yin and Yang (Yin Yang Lun) 二・陰陽論

It is seldom heard that he who discusses striking, also discussed Qi. About the Qi, it is mastered as one but can be divided into two. What are these two? They are inhaling and exhaling. The inhalation and exhalation are the Yin and Yang. The striking cannot (be done) without moving and calmness. The Qi cannot (exist) without inhaling and exhaling. Inhalation is Yin and exhalation is Yang. The one which is calm is Yin and the one which is moving is Yang. Raising up is Yang and sinking downward is Yin. When Yang Qi is rising up it becomes Yang, and when Yang Qi is being transported downward it becomes Yin. When Yin Qi is being transported downward it becomes Yin, and when Yin Qi is being transported upward it becomes Yang. This is the discrimination of Yin and Yang.

嘗有世之論捶者者，而兼論氣者矣。夫氣主於一，可分為
二。所謂二者，即呼吸也。呼吸即陰陽也。捶不能無動
靜，氣不能無呼吸。吸則為陰，呼則為陽。主乎靜者為
陰，主乎動者為陽。上升為陽，下降為陰。陽氣上升為
陽，陽氣下行為陰。陰氣下行而為陰，陰氣上行即為陽，
此陰陽之分也。

At the time when Yue, Fei was writing these theses, few martial artists were using Qigong to improve their martial abilities. Qi can energize the muscles to reach their maximum potential, and it can also raise the spirit of vitality to a higher level. Through Qi you can be calm, and through Qi you can be excited. Through the behavior or action of Qi, your emotional state, thinking, and movements can be distinguished into Yin and Yang. Generally, Yin is the seed of Yang and Yang is the blossom of Yin. Yin is for storage and Yang is for manifestation. Yin is sunken and Yang is raised. Yin is steady and calm and Yang is excited and powerful. All of these manifestations of Yin and Yang are generated through inhalation and exhalation. Inhalation and exhalation are considered the strategy in Chinese Qigong. Proper inhalation and exhalation techniques can adjust the Yin and Yang of the body. Therefore, to be a proficient martial artist you must know these two strategies for controlling the state of your body.

What is meant (by) clean and muddy? The one that rises up to the top is clean and the one descending downward is muddy. The clean Qi rises upward and the dirty Qi sinks downward. The clean one is Yang and the dirty one is Yin. The important (thing) is that Yang should be used to nourish Yin. Generally speaking, they (i.e., Yin and Yang Qi) are united as (one) Qi, if divided, they are distinguished as Yin and Yang. Qi cannot be without Yin and Yang, and it is just like man cannot be (alive) without having movement and calmness, the nose cannot be without inhalation and exhalation, and the mouth cannot be (with) no exiting and entering. This is the unchangeable theory of natural cycling. However, though Qi can be divided into two, in fact, it is one. Those who like to study this should be careful not to restrict this (theory).

何謂清濁？升而上者為清，降而下者為濁。清氣上升，
濁氣下降。清者為陽，濁者為陰。而要之，陽以滋陰，
渾而言之統為氣，分而言之為陰陽。氣不能無陰陽，即
所謂人不能無動靜，鼻不能無呼吸，口不能無出入，此
即對待循環不易之理也。然則氣分為二，而實在於一。
有志於斯途者，慎勿以是為拘拘焉。

In order to make your mind calm so that you can think clearly, you must sink your "muddy" Qi to the Lower Dan Tian. This refers to the Fire Qi, which can make your body too Yang and your mind overexcited, unstable, unclear, and confused.

Clean Qi refers to Water Qi, which makes your body Yin and calms down emotional confusion. This makes it possible for your judgement to be accurate and neutral. This seems to indicate that Yin and Yang are two distinct things, but, in fact, Yin and Yang cannot be separated. Yin is the root and the seed of Yang, but it also needs Yang to nourish it so it can grow. Without the nourishment of Yang, Yin will not grow and gradually derive into Yang. Out of Yang is produced the seed (Yin). Also, without Yin, the Yang will have nothing to grow from.

Although Qi can be divided into Yin and Yang states, in fact, there is only one kind of Qi. Yin and Yang are the result of the manifestation of Qi in the body. If you are bound and restricted by this theory, then it is dead and not alive. The fact is, Yin and Yang are relative, not absolute. This is important for you to realize if you want to understand Yin-Yang theory and apply it properly.

3. Thesis of the Three Sections (San Jie Lun) 三‧三節論

Qi is the root of the entire body and the sections of the body do not have definite places/positions. What are called the "three sections" are the top, middle, and bottom. For the body, the head is the top section, the body is the middle section, and the legs are the bottom section. If (we) talk about (only) the top section, then the crown is the top section, the nose is the middle section, and the tongue (Haidi) is the bottom section. If (we) talk about the middle section, then the chest is the top section, the abdomen is the middle section, and the Dan Tian is the bottom section. If (we) talk about the bottom section, the feet are the ending section, the knees are the middle section, and the hips are the root section. If (we) talk about the arms, the hands are the ending section, the elbows are the middle section, and the shoulders are the root section. If (we) talk about the hands, the fingers are the ending section, the palms are the middle section, and the roots of the palms (i.e., near wrists) are the root section. From this, (we) do not have to talk more about feet (i.e., give more examples).

夫氣本諸身，而身之節無定處。三節者，上、中、下也。以身言之：頭為上節，身為中節，腿為下節。以上節言之：天庭為上節，鼻為中節，海底為下節。以中節言之：胸為上節，腹為中節，丹田為下節。以下節言之：足為梢節，膝為中節，胯為根節。以肱言之：手為梢節，肘為中節，肩為根節。以手言之：指為梢節，掌為中節，掌根為根節。觀於是，而足不必論矣。

If you look at your body from the point of view of Qi, the body should not be divided. This is because the Qi in the body is continuous and threaded together into one. However, if you look at your body from the physical perspective, then you can divide it into three sections in many different ways. This is done solely for the convenience of discussion. Other than this, however, your mind should not be restricted by these divisions. Your body should act as a unit, and should not be broken into parts. Haidi (海底) means "sea bottom" which implies the tongue.

However, from the head to the feet, all have three sections. The important (point) is that if there is not a distinguishing into three sections, then the meaning cannot be clear. Because (if) the top section is not clear, there is no dependence and no origin. (If) the middle section is not clear, then the entire body is void. (If) the bottom section is not clear, then you will fall by yourself. How can we ignore them? As to how the Qi starts to move, there is nothing but the end section must move, the middle section follows, and the root section urges. However, all of these discussions are because (we) divide (the body) into sections and talk about them. If we talk about when they are all combined, then from the top of the head to the bottom of the feet, the four limbs and hundreds of bones, all in one section, how can they be divided into three sections? Furthermore, how can we again divide each section of these three sections into another three sections?

然則自頂至足，莫不各有三節。要之，若無三節之分，
即無著意之處。蓋上節不明，無依無宗，中節不明，渾
身是空，下節不明，自家吃跌，顧可忽乎哉。至於氣之
發動，要皆梢節動，中節隨，根節催之而已。然此猶是
節節而分言之者也；若夫合言之，則上至頭頂，下至足
底，四肢百骸，總為一節，夫何三節之有哉？又何三節
中之各有三節云乎哉？

You can see from the previous paragraph that there are many ways to divide your body into three sections. The sole purpose for this is to make the meaning (i.e., explanation) clear. For example, if the head (top section) is not clear, then your thinking will not be clear and ideas will not be generated. Ideas are the main motivation of movement. If the chest and the waist (middle section) are not clearly connected to the head (top section) and to the legs (bottom section), then this center portion of the body will be missing, and the body will lose the physical center of its movements. Finally, if you do not have a clear understanding of the meaning (i.e., purpose and function) of the legs (bottom section), then you will lose your root and foundation, and even though you have a clear idea of what you want to do and can control your torso, your movements will not be smooth and efficient.

For each movement, the secret of starting the Qi is your Yi. When your Yi generates the idea for a movement, the Qi will be led immediately to the end section. This starts the movement of the end section. The middle section naturally follows, and the root section urges the movement. This concept is different from how Jin is manifested in Taijiquan. In Taijiquan, Jin is generated first in the root section, directed by the middle section, and finally manifested in the end section. The reason for this difference is that in Taijiquan the body is like a whip, soft and very relaxed. When the mind generates an idea, the legs first generate the power (shoulder), the power is directed by the waist (wrist), and manifested in the fingers (tip of the whip). However, in Xingyiquan, the body acts like rattan. Though flexible, it is still hard. Therefore, when the Yi is generated on the target, the tip can move first, and the power is pushed from the body and the root section.

4. Thesis of the Four Extremities (Si Shao Lun) 四 · 四梢論

(Now let us) try, in addition to discussing the body and the Qi, to discuss the extremities. The extremities are the surplus ends of the body. Those who talk about the body have never mentioned these since the beginning, and those who talk about the Qi have also seldom discussed them. Striking is (generated) from the internal and emitted to the outside, and thus the Qi is (generated) from the body and reaches to the extremities. Therefore, (if) the application of Qi does not originate from the body, then (this application) is void and not solid. (If the application of Qi) does not manifest in every extremity, though solid, it is still void. How can (we) not talk about the extremities? However, (we have mentioned) only the extremities of the physical body and have not mentioned the extremities of the Qi.

> 試於論身論氣之外，而進論乎梢者焉。夫梢者，身之餘
> 緒也；言身者初不及此，言氣者亦所罕論。捶以內而發
> 外，氣由身而達梢，故氣之用不本諸身，則虛而不實，
> 不形諸梢，則實而仍虛，梢亦烏可不講。然子特身之梢
> 耳，而猶未及乎氣之梢也。

The four extremities are not the limbs, which is what one would ordinarily think. Instead they are the hair, the tongue, the nails, and the teeth. Chinese doctors frequently diagnose patients by examining the condition of these extremities. Chinese medicine and Qigong believe that these four extremities will be healthy only when your Qi is circulating smoothly and properly in your body. Therefore, in Xingyiquan it is believed that you should learn how to lead the Qi to them, for only then will you have proven that your Qi is abundant and circulating without stagnation. Only then are you able to manifest your Jin to the maximum. Therefore, Xingyiquan emphasizes that the Qi is originated internally and must be connected and manifested externally in these four extremities.

> *What are the four extremities? The hair is one. Because the hair does not belong to one of the Five Phases and is not related to the four limbs, it seems that (it) is not worth discussing. However, the hair is the ending of the blood and the blood is the ocean of Qi. Even though we do not use the hair to discuss Qi, (we still) cannot ignore the blood (when we discuss) the generation of Qi. (If we) cannot ignore the blood, then (we) cannot but also be concerned with the hair. (When) the hair is (strong enough) to shoot up the hat, (the Qi) in the blood ending is sufficient. Others such as the tongue is the ending of the meat (muscles) and the meat is the Qi bag (i.e., capable of storing Qi). (If) the Qi cannot be manifested in the ending of the meat, then there is not enough quantity of Qi to fill up (the muscles). Therefore, the tongue should urge (i.e., push against) the teeth, then (the Qi) in the meat ending will be enough.*

四梢唯何？髮其一也。夫髮之所係，不列於五形，無關
於四體，似不足論矣；然髮為血之梢，血為氣之海，縱
不必本諸髮以論氣，要不能離乎血而生氣，不離乎血，
即不得不兼及乎髮。髮欲沖冠，血梢足矣。其他如舌為
肉梢，而肉為氣囊，氣不能形諸肉之梢，即無以充其氣
之量，故必舌催齒，而後肉梢足矣。

The first extremity is the hair. According to Chinese medicine, the hair is close-ly related to the blood, which is a carrier of Qi. The blood cells need Qi in order to function. They also, it is now believed, act like batteries and store Qi, releasing it to the parts of the body that require it. In Chinese medicine, Qi and blood are fre-quently used together as one word (Qi Xue, 氣血).

When your blood cells are healthy and are able to store an abundance of Qi, they will carry Qi to the surface of your skin and stimulate hair growth. When your spir-it is excited, this Qi will give the hair an electrical charge, and it will stand up like a cat's does when it is excited.

In the same way, the tongue is considered to have a close connection with the muscles. Muscles are like a storage bag for Qi. When you exercise the same muscle repeatedly, the Qi and blood will gather in that muscle. When you relax after fin-ishing your exercise, the stored Qi will be released to the outside or will re-enter the Qi channels in the body. In order to make your techniques powerful and effective, you must be able to lead the Qi to the muscles efficiently in order to energize them to the maximum. Since the tongue is the ending or extremity of the muscles, if you are able to lead Qi to the tongue, surely you have already effectively led Qi to the muscles.

> As to the ending of the bones, it is the teeth. The ending of the tendons is the nails. Qi is generated from the bones, which are connected to the tendons. (If the Qi) cannot reach the teeth, it means (the Qi) cannot reach the ending of the tendons (either). (If you) desire to have plenty (of Qi), then it cannot be done unless (your) teeth are able to break the tendons and the nails are able to penetrate the bones. If (you) are able to do this, (then the Qi) of the four extremities is suffi-cient. When (the Qi) of the four extremities is sufficient, the Qi (in your body) will be plenty automatically. In this case, how can it be still void (i.e., the Qi be deficient) and not solid (i.e., the physical body not be strong), or though solid still void?

至於骨梢者，齒也。筋梢者，指甲也。氣生於骨，而聯
於筋，不及乎齒，即未及乎筋之梢，而欲足乎爾者，要
非齒欲斷筋，甲欲透骨，不能也。果能如此，則四梢足
矣。四梢足而氣亦自足矣。豈復有虛而不實，實而仍虛
者乎。

Qi has to fill the whole body. If you try to make each ending stronger than the others, you will end up strengthening them all equally, and your whole body will be strong. In this case, how could you have abundant Qi and not have a strong body?

5. Thesis of the Five Phases (Wu Xing Lun) 五·五形論

Today when (we) talk about striking, (first we) discuss the postures. When (we) talk about the postures, (first we) discuss Qi. Man has five viscera which therefore form the shape. That is (because) from the five viscera, the Qi is born. (Therefore) the five viscera are really the original bearers of human nature (i.e., life) and the source of growing Qi. (These five viscera are) named heart, liver, spleen, lungs, and kidneys. The heart is (classified as) Fire and has the appearance of flaming upward. The liver is (classified as) Wood and has the shape of curved and straight. The spleen is (classified as) Earth and has the feeling of solid and sincere. The lungs are (classified as) Metal and have the capability of initiating changes (in the body). The kidneys are (classified as) Water and have the talent of moistening the lower body. This is the meaning of the five viscera, and they must be coordinated accurately with the Qi so that they are able to cooperate with each other.

今夫捶以言勢，勢以言氣，人得五臟以成形，即由五臟而生氣。五臟實為生性之源，生氣之本，而名心、肝、脾、肺、腎是也。心為火，而有炎上之象；肝為木，而有曲直之形；脾為土，而有敦厚之勢；肺為金，而有從革之能；腎為水，而有潤下之功；此乃五臟之義，而必準之於氣者，以其各有所配合焉。

When we talk about striking we usually first discuss the correct postures, which most efficiently protect the body and most effectively manifest Jin. Then, when we analyze the postures for manifesting Jin, we have to begin discussing Qi. Finally, when we discuss the Qi, we must first understand where the Qi comes from. Qi comes from the conversion of Essence (Jing, 精). Essence includes the food and air Essence (Post-Birth Essence), and the Essence which you inherit from your parents (Original Essence or Pre-Birth Essence)(Yuan Jing, 元精). Interested readers please see Dr. Yang's book, *The Root of Chinese Qigong*, for a detailed discussion. Your five Yin viscera (heart, lungs, liver, kidneys, and spleen) are the organs responsible for converting the Essence into Qi and distributing it to your entire body. Therefore, it says that Qi originates from the five viscera. It is this generation and distribution of Qi which is responsible for your being alive, and also for the growth of your individual and human nature.

Chinese medicine and Qigong classify the viscera according to the principle of the Five Phases. According to their character, function, and mutual relationships, the viscera are classified as Fire (heart), Wood (liver), Earth (spleen), Metal (lungs), and Water (kidneys).

This is why those who talk about martial affairs must not separate from them. The chest and diaphragm is the position of the lung primary Qi channel and (they) cover all other viscera. Therefore, when (the Qi in) the lung primary channel moves, all other viscera cannot be calm. The heart is between the two nipples and enwrapped and protected by the lungs. Underneath the lungs and above the stomach is the location of the heart primary Qi channel. The heart is the king of

Fire, and once it moves all other primary ministerial Fires will naturally follow. Between the two flanks, left is the liver and right is the spleen. On the fourteenth section of the spine are the kidneys. These are the positions of the five viscera. However, all these five viscera are linked with the back spine and connected with the kidneys' essence. As to the waist, it is the home position of the two kidneys. (They) are the first (in importance) among the pre-heaven (organs) and especially are the origin and root of all other viscera. Therefore, when the kidney Water is sufficient, then Metal, Wood, Water, Fire, and Earth will have the opportunity to (create) life. These are the positions of the five viscera.

此所以論武事者，要不能離乎斯也。胸膈為肺經之位，
而為諸臟之華蓋，故肺經動而諸臟不能靜。兩乳之中為
心，而肺包護之，肺之下，胃之上，心經之位也。心為
君火，動而相火無不奉合焉。而兩腎之間，左為肝，右
為脾，背脊十四骨節，皆為腎，此固五臟之位。然五臟
之係，皆係於背脊，通於腎髓，故為腎。至於腰，則兩
腎之本位，而為先天之第一，尤為諸臟之根源。故腎水
足，而金、木、水、火、土咸有生機，此乃五臟之位也。

The location of the organs is given from the perspective of someone looking at a person from the front. Three of the Yin organs are especially important. The first is the lungs, which take in air Essence and convert it into Qi, which is distributed throughout the body by the blood. Therefore, once the lungs are in action, the other four viscera cannot be calm. Then, the heart is the residence of the emotional Fire. When this Fire starts (when the emotional mind is activated), all other viscera will also become fiery (excited). Finally, the most important of the viscera is the kidneys. They are the residence of the Pre-Birth Essence (Yuan Jing, Original Essence)(元精). Original Essence is the source of Water Qi, which cools the body's Fire and therefore balances the Yin and Yang. The Yin and Yang must be balanced and interact harmoniously for you to be healthy. You can see that the kidneys' Water is ultimately the most important element in regulating the conditions of the other four organs and effecting the balance of Yin and Yang.

In addition, the five viscera existing internally have their definite positions. Manifested (externally) on the body, they (i.e., the manifestations) also have their special positions. They are (manifested on) the neck, the top of head, the brain, the bones, the back, and the kidneys (i.e., ears). The two ears are also (related to) the kidneys, the two lips and two cheeks are (related to) the spleen. Two hairs (i.e., the hair on the two sides of the head) are the lungs. The forehead is the leader of the six Yang organs and gathers the Essence of the five viscera (i.e., five Yin organs) and actually is the main master of the head and face and is the governor of the entire body.

且五臟之存於內者，各有其定位，而具於身者，亦自有
專屬，領、頂、腦、骨、背、腎是也。兩耳亦為腎，兩
唇、兩腮、皆脾也。兩髮則為肺。天庭為六陽之首，而
萃五臟之精華，實為頭面之主腦，不啻一身之座督矣。

In addition to having definite locations inside the body, the five viscera have particular locations on the outside of the body where their condition is manifested. Most of the these manifestations are shown on the head. For example, the two ears are related to the two kidneys, the lips and cheeks are linked to the spleen. The hair on the sides of the head is related to the lungs. However, the most important of all is the forehead, especially above the eye bridge (i.e., the third eye)(Tian Yan, 天眼), which is considered to be the residence of the spirit and is called the Upper Dan Tian (Shang Dan Tian, 上丹田) in Chinese Qigong. The spirit is the center of one's being, and governs the Qi distribution in the entire body, especially the manifestation of the six Yang channels.

> *The Yintang, (is) the key place or the Stomach Qi of Yang Brightness. When the human nature (Xing) starts at the Tianting, its functioning is approached from here. The Qi generated and developed (here) is able to reach the six Yangs from the kidneys and it (i.e., the Yintang) is really the main key place of the Tianting. Two eyes are both (related to) the liver. Studied in more detail, the bottom (of the eyes) is the spleen and the top is the stomach. The big corner is for the heart channel and the small corner is for the small intestines. The white (of the eyes) means the lungs and the black is the liver. The pupil is the kidneys and is actually the Essence gathering of the five viscera. (Therefore, the eyes are) not only especially related to the liver.*

> 印堂者，陽明胃氣之衝，天庭性起，機由此達，生發之
> 氣，由腎而達於六陽，實為天庭之樞機也。兩目皆為肝，
> 而究之下包為脾，上包為胃，大角為心經，小角為小腸，
> 白則為肺，黑則為肝，瞳則為腎，實為五臟精華所聚，
> 而不得專謂之肝也。

The Yintang (印堂) is the space between the eyebrows. The Stomach Qi channel (Figure A-1) ends in this area. Tianting (天庭) is the name for the forehead, which is the residence of the spirit, which governs the six Yang channels and is also the center of your human nature. If the spirit here is raised to a high]eve], the Water Qi generated from the kidneys can be effectively and smoothly distributed. The eyes are related to the liver. In the last few years Chinese medicine has found correspondences between parts of the eyes and all twelve internal organs (Figure A-2). This is discussed in Dr. Yang's book, *Qigong for Health and Martial Arts*.

> *The nose is (related to) the lungs, the two cheeks are (also related to) the kidneys, the front of the ear doors are (related to) the Gall Bladder, and the high bones behind the ears are also (related to) the kidneys. The nose is the Earth Center and is the source of the birth and nourishment of the million objects. (The nose) is actually the master of the center Qi. The Renzhong is the meeting (place) of blood and Qi, (it) thrusts upward into the Yintang and reaches to the Tianting; it is also the most important place. Under the two lips is the Chengjiang and underneath the Chengjiang is the Dihe. (They) correspond to the Tianting and also relate to the kidney channel.*

The Stomach Chi Channel

Yintang (M-NH-3)

Figure A-1. Yintang cavity

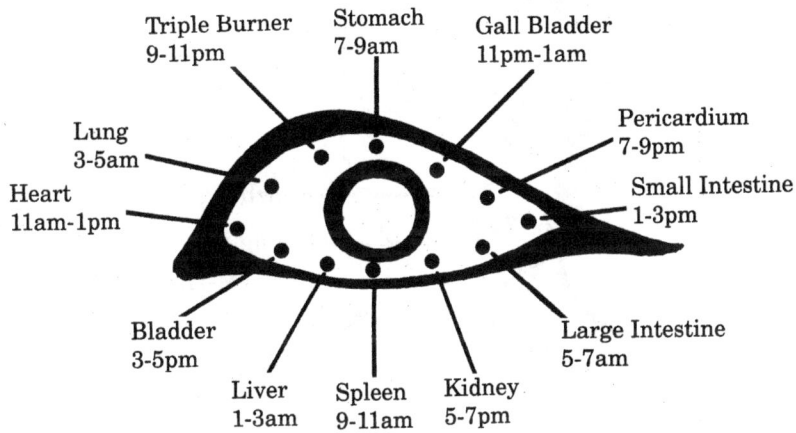

Triple Burner
9-11pm

Stomach
7-9am

Gall Bladder
11pm-1am

Lung
3-5am

Pericardium
7-9pm

Heart
11am-1pm

Small Intestine
1-3pm

Bladder
3-5pm

Large Intestine
5-7am

Liver
1-3am

Spleen
9-11am

Kidney
5-7pm

Figure A-2. Correspondence between parts of the eyes and the twelve primary channels

鼻孔為肺，兩頤為腎，耳門之前為膽經，耳後之高骨，
亦腎也。鼻為中央之土，萬物資生之源，實為中氣之主
也。人中為血氣之會，上沖印堂，達於天庭，亦為至要
之所。兩唇之下為承漿，承漿之下為地閣，上與天庭相
應，亦腎經位也。

Since the nose is used to take in air, which is necessary for life, it is considered to be the "Earth Center." The nose is therefore the main source for obtaining Post-Birth Qi. Renzhong (Gv-26)(人中) is the spot under the nose which is the junction of the Stomach channel and the Governing Vessel. According to this document, Renzhong (Figure A-3) is considered the meeting place of blood and Qi. From here the Qi is thrust upward to the Yintang (M-NH-3)(印堂) and the top of the forehead. Underneath the lips is Chengjiang (Co-24)(承漿), and under Chengjiang is Dihe (M-HN-19)(地閣). Though the above mentioned cavities belong to the Stomach channel, they still reflect the condition of the kidneys.

The head and neck are the pathway to the five viscera and the main gathering place of blood and Qi. The front is the entering and exiting path of food and air and the rear is the ascending and descending way of kidney Qi. The liver Qi is thus spinning to the left and the spleen Qi is spinning to the right. Their relations are most important and are the key points of (Qi distribution in) the entire body. (Between) the two nipples is the liver and (between) the two shoulders are the lungs, (between) the two elbows are the kidneys, (between) the two shoulders on the back is the spleen. The ten fingers are (connected to) the heart, liver, spleen, lungs, and kidneys. The knees and the calves are all (related to) the kidneys. The bottoms of the two feet are the important (places) of the kidneys and the Yongquan are the cavities of the kidneys.

Figure A-3. Renzhong, Chengjiang, and Dige cavities

— Renzhong (Gv-26)

— Chengjiang (Co-24)

— Dihe (M-HN-19)

領、頂、頸、項者，五臟之道途，氣血之總會，前為食
氣出入之道，後為腎氣升降之途，肝氣由之而左旋，脾
氣由之而右旋，其係更重，而為周身之要領。兩乳為肝，
兩肩為肺，兩肘為腎，四肢為脾，兩肩背膊皆為脾，而
十指則為心、肝、脾、肺、腎是也。膝與脛，皆腎也。
兩腳根為腎之要，湧泉為腎穴。

According to Chinese medicine, in the front of the body is the tripleburner, which is divided into the upper burner, middle burner, and lower burner. The upper burner converts air Essence into Qi, while the other two burners handle food Essence, converting it through biochemical reaction into Qi. Therefore, the Fire Qi (which is created from air and food) is generated in the front of the body. However, there is also another Qi, classified as Water Qi. Water Qi is generated from the conversion of the Original Essence which you inherit from your parents and which is stored in the kidneys. When Water Qi is produced, it rises to nourish the brain, and also moves downward to the Lower Dan Tian, which is its residence. Fire and Water Qi also nourish the liver and spleen to keep them functioning.

Generally, how the body is related (to the organs), those places which are convex are (related to) the heart, those concave are (related to) the lungs, those places where the bone is exposed (i.e., shallow) are (related to) the kidneys, the tendons junction places are (related to) the liver, and those (places where) the meat is thick are (related to) the spleen. Looking at them from the (point of view of the) Yi, the heart is like a fiery tiger, the liver is like an arrow, the spleen with the unlimited strength of Qi and Li. The distribution of the liver channel is the most variable spiritually (i.e., sensitive), the movement of the kidneys' Qi is fast like the wind. When (these are) applied to the body such as the application of Qi channels, (when we talk about) the places in the entire body which are related to these channels, ultimately they cannot be (understood) without having the meaning (i.e., Yi). Therefore, people studying (this) should comprehend (these) by themselves. (These) cannot be done through pen and ink. As to the (relation of) production, conquest, and derivation, though there is some other discussion already, if (we) study their key points, then there is a total comprehension automatically. The Five Phases and the hundreds of (parts of the) body, after all, are one unit. The four bodies and the three centers are combined into one. Why do we have to pay attention to every channel and every branch or section of the body?

大約身之所係，凸者為心，窩者為肺，骨之露處皆為腎，
筋之聯處皆為肝，肉之厚處皆為脾。象其意，心如猛虎，
肝如箭，脾氣力大甚無窮，肝經之位最靈變，腎氣之動
快如風。其為用也，用其經，舉凡身之所屬於某經者，
終不能無意焉，是在當局者自為體認，而非筆墨所能為
者也。至於生克治化，雖別有論，而究其要領，自有統
會，五行百體，總為一元，四體三心，合為一氣，奚必
昭昭於某一經絡，而支支節節言之哉。

This paragraph continues to discuss the relationship of the external manifestation and the internal organs. In order to comprehend the real meaning (i.e., the deeper purpose) of each organ, you must also feel how they behave. For example, the heart can act like a fierce tiger, the liver can be as simple and calm as wood. The spleen is like the earth which is able to offer unlimited Li (力)(i.e., muscular power) and Qi, and the kidneys' Qi must flow smoothly and fluidly like the wind. When you combine these meanings in your feelings, you will be able to reach a deep comprehension of the five viscera. Among these five, although they have the relationships of mutual production and conquest, from the point of view of Qi, there is only one. The four bodies here mean the head, the body, the arms, and the legs. The three centers are the center pointing downward from the head, the center pointing upward from the feet, and the center directing inward from the arms.

---

6. Thesis of the Six Combinations (Liu He Lun) 六 · 六合論

Xin combines with Yi, Yi combines with Qi, and Qi combines with Li are the three internal combinations. Hands combine with feet, elbows combine with knees, and shoulders combine with hips are the three external combinations. These are called "Liu He" (the six combinations). The left hand combines with the right foot, the left elbow combines with the right knee, the left shoulder combines with the right hip. The same for the other side. Then, the head combines with the hands, the hands combine with the body, and the body combines with the stepping. (These) cannot be thought not to be the external combinations. The heart combines with the eyes, the liver combines with the tendons, the spleen combines with the meat, the lungs combine with the body, and the kidneys combine with the bones. (These) cannot be thought not to be the internal combinations. (In this case), how can there be only six combinations? They are divided only for discussion. In all, (when) one place moves, nowhere does not move; (when) one place combines, no place is not combined. (Then) the five shapes and hundreds of bones will all be useful.

心與意合，意與氣合，氣與力合，內三合也。手與足合，
肘與膝合，肩與胯合，外三合也。此為六合。左手與右
足相合，左肘與右膝相合，左肩與右胯相合，右之與左
亦然。以及頭與手合，手與身合，身與步合，孰非外合；
心與眼合，肝與筋合，脾與肉合，肺與身合，腎與骨合，
孰非內合。豈但六合而已哉。然此特分而言之也。總之
一動而無不動，一合而無不合。五形百骸，悉用其中矣。

In Chinese culture, the Xin (心) is considered the mind generated from the emotions, and the Yi (意) is the mind generated from the wise and clear judgement. The emotional mind is able to make you excited and the wisdom mind is able to calm you down. When you train Xingyiquan, you must learn to use your wisdom mind to govern your emotional mind, then they can be united. When you have this combination, your Yi can be concentrated and can effectively lead the Qi so that the

Yi and Qi can be combined. Once your Qi and Yi combine and the Qi can be led effectively by the Yi to the muscles to energize them, then the muscular power (Li, 力) can be raised to a higher level and thus the Qi and the Li are combined. All these three combinations are internal and cannot be seen.

Externally, there are also three combinations. These are the hands and the feet combine, the elbows and the knees combine, and the shoulders and the hips combine. Other than the above six combinations, other portions of the body should also be related and combined. In addition, the internal and the external should also be combined. Only when you have achieved all of these combination can your entire body act as one unit both externally and internally. The-five shapes (Wu Xing, 五形) means the head and the four limbs.

---

7. Thesis of the Seven Advancings (Qi Jin Lun) 七 · 七進論

The head is the leader of the six Yangs and is also the master of the entire body. The five sensing organs and hundreds of bones do not but rely on it. Therefore, the head cannot but advance. The hands move first, and their foundation and root are in the shoulders. If the shoulders do not advance, then the hands will hesitate and not advance. Therefore, it is important that the shoulders must advance. Qi is gathered in the Zhongwan cavity and the key is in the waist; when the waist does not advance, then the Qi is weak and not solid. Therefore, it is important that the waist must advance.

> 頭為六陽之首，而為周身之主，五官百骸，莫不惟此是
> 賴。故頭不可不進也。手為先行，根基在膊，膊不進，
> 而手則卻而不前矣。此所以膊貴於進也。氣聚中脘，機
> 關在腰，腰不進，而氣則餒而不實也。此所以腰貴於進
> 也。

The head here means the idea and the raised spirit. Since they are the origin of any action, the head is the master of the entire body. Therefore, in a fight, you must generate your idea and raise up your spirit first. If you are afraid, your mind will not be clear and your spirit will be weak. In this case, how can you win the fight? In the actual movement, the hands should not hesitate. Since the shoulders are the root and the foundation of the hands, the shoulders must also advance. If the shoulders do not advance, how can you expect the hands to advance?

Qi gathers in the Lower Dan Tian (下丹田) near the Zhongwan (Co-12)(中脘) and Qihai (Co-6)(氣海) cavities on the front of the waist (Figure A-4). Therefore, the stored Qi must also advance. If it cannot advance, then you will not have abundant Qi to energize the entire body and raise up your fighting spirit.

Yi is threaded throughout the entire body, and the movements (depend) on the stepping. (If) the stepping is not forward, then the Yi is in vain and cannot do anything. Therefore, the stepping is important in advancing. Then, when attack-

ing the left, the right must be advanced, and when attacking the right, the left must be advanced. These are the seven advancings. They are not what is called the advancing in touching the ground (i.e., moving forward). To conclude their importance, before advancing, the entire body may not have the Yi connection and be related to each other, (however) once talking about advancing, then the entire body does not have the appearance of delaying and hesitation.

意貫周身，運動在步，步不進而意則堂然無能為矣。此
所以步必取其進也。以及上左必須進右，上右必須進左，
其為七進，執非所以著力之地歟。而要之，未及其進，
合周身而毫無關動之意，一言其進，統全體而俱無抽扯
游移之形。

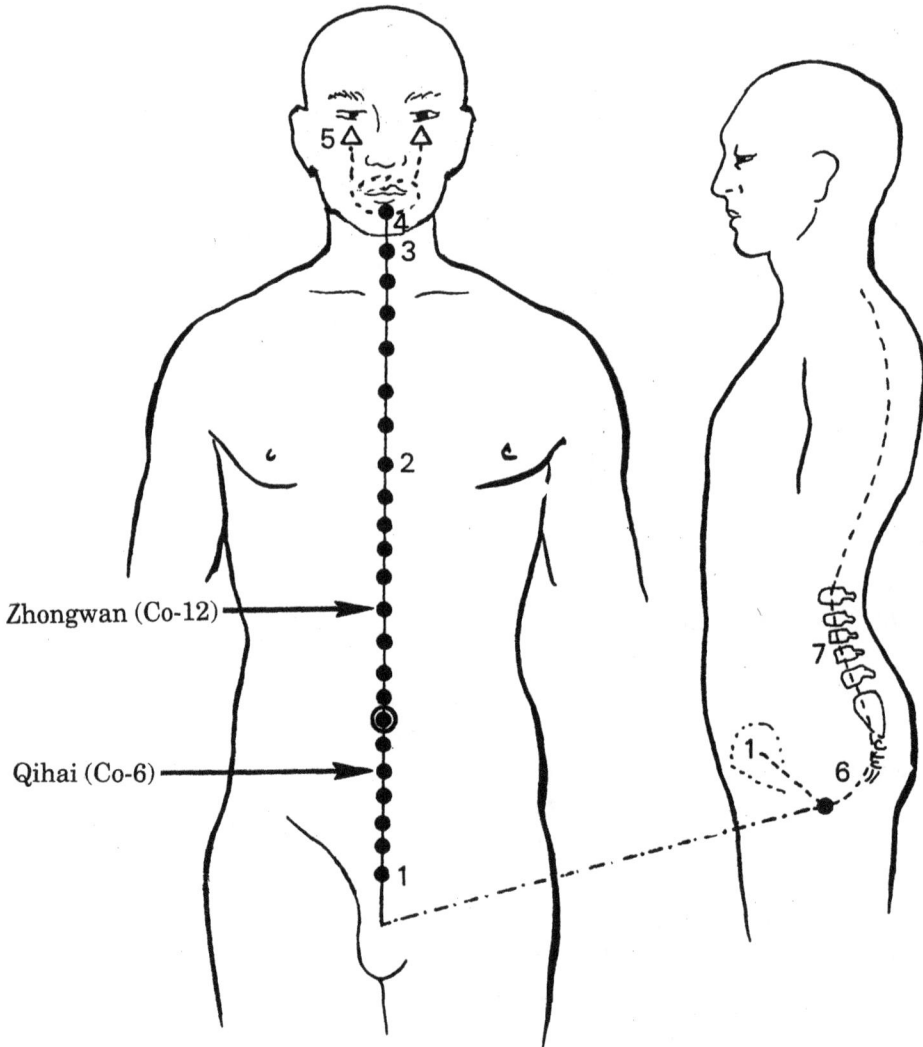

Figure A-4. Zhongwan and Qihai cavities

In addition to the above four advances, the other three are the stepping and the two sides. If you have the Yi of advancing but your legs are not obeying your mind, then everything will be in vain. Strategywise, you must also be skillful in advancing sideways. Left and right can be either substantial or insubstantial. If you are able to grasp the tricks of these seven advancings, you will gain the advantage in battle.

---

8. Thesis of the Body's Maneuvers (Shen Fa Lun) 八・身法論

What are the body's maneuvers? Simply, (they are) Zong (straight forward), Heng (sideways), Gao (moving high), Di (moving low), Jin (advancing), Tui (retreating), Fan (reversing), and Ce (beware of the flank). Zong is releasing the posture forward and not returning. Heng is to enwrap the (opponent's) Li, opening up the way which cannot be resisted. Gao is to extend the body, and the body has the tendency to grow (high). Di is to press down the body and make the body have the shape of drilling and seizing. When it should be forward, then forward. Bounce the body and straight forward bravely. When you should retreat, then retreat. Lead the Qi back and convert the posture into yielding.

身法為何？縱橫高低進退反側而已。縱則放其勢，一往
而不返。橫則裹其力，開拓而莫阻。高則揚其身，而身
若有增長之勢。低則抑其身，而身若有鑽捉之形，當進
則進，殫其身而勇往直冲；當退則退，領其氣而回轉伏
勢。

Zong (縱) in Chinese means vertical and directly forward or backward, and has the feeling of moving freely. When you apply these ideas to Xingyiquan, it means free to get in on the opponent while keeping your body upright. Heng (橫) in Chinese means sideways, and has the feeling of forcing your way in violently. Therefore, when this word is applied in Xingyiquan, it means to force or to push obstacles to the side. In order to clear the way in effectively, Heng also has the meaning of wrapping, coiling, sticking, neutralizing, and many other techniques. Without these key techniques, Heng would only be a sideward block. Simply put, Heng means to enwrap the opponent's power and lead it to the side.

Gao (高) means high or rising. In Xingyiquan it means the raising of the body in coordination with the drilling of a hand or leg. Di (低) means low or falling. In Xingyiquan, it means to lower the body with a curling motion. Jin (進) means to enter or to advance. In Xingyiquan, it means to step or to charge straight forward. Tui (退) means to retreat or to get out of a disadvantageous position. Fan (反) means to reverse or to turn around. In Xingyiquan, it means to beware of the rear and to turn your body around. Naturally, you must also know Ce (側), which means to beware of the sides so that you can dodge an attack, or you may enter from the side to attack the opponent.

As to turning the body and beware of the rear, the rear is the front. When I beware of the left and right, (this will) make nobody dare to resist me from the left or the right. (You) should not be inhibited. First, (you) must inspect the opponent's strong and weak (points), (then) skillfully apply my (i.e., your) key tricks (i.e., techniques), sometimes suddenly forward and suddenly sideways. Forward and sideways are changeable following the situation and (you) cannot set a general rule to follow. There is suddenly high and suddenly low, they can be switched anytime, (you) cannot be stubborn in the rules and talk about (the situation). When it is time to advance, then (you) cannot retreat, if (you) retreat, then the Qi strength is weakened. When it is time to retreat, then retreat to prepare for an advance.

> 至於反身顧後，後即前也。側顧左右，使左右無敢當我，
> 而要非拘拘焉為之也。必先察人之強弱，運吾之機關，
> 有忽縱而忽橫，縱橫因勢而變遷，不可一概而推。有忽
> 高而忽低，高低隨時可以轉移，不可執格而論。時而宜
> 進，故不可退而餒其氣；時而可退，即當以退而鼓其進。

When you are in a battle, you are not fighting against only one enemy. Very often you will be attacked from the rear. Therefore, you must beware of the rear and consider it as important as the front. In this case, there is no difference between where the front is and where the rear is. You should treat the sides the same way. When you are in a fight, you must beware of the four directions and be capable of attacking in any direction. Your strategy and techniques are alive and can be applied to any situation. In this case, the enemy will not be able to figure you out and he will not dare to resist you. In order to achieve this marvelous ability to move, your strategy and techniques should not be restricted by conventional, conservative rules or principles.

(Therefore), advance is for advancing and even retreating, it also relies on (retreating) for advance. If you turn the body to beware of the rear, (even when you) beware of the rear, still never feel it is the rear. When you beware of the left and right, the left and right are never felt to be left and right. In all, the key is in the eyes, and the change is from the heart, then when the key is held, it is applied to the body. When the body is moving forward, it does not need an order, the four limbs are forward. When the body is retreating, then hundreds of skeleton bones are all in their positions scientifically. (In this case) how can we not talk about the body's maneuvers?

> 是進固進也，即退，而亦實以賴其進。若反身顧後，顧
> 其後而亦不覺其為後，側顧左右，而左右亦不覺其為左
> 右矣。總之，機關在眼，變通在心，而握其要者，則本
> 諸身。身而前，則四體不令而行矣；身而卻，則百骸莫
> 不冥然而處矣。身法顧可置而不論乎。

When you have reached this high level of fighting, when you advance you are advancing, and even when you are retreating you are still advancing. Retreating is only a strategy for advancing. You should train yourself to be capable of fighting in every direction. Then there is no difference between front and rear and left and right.

Through careful inspection with your eyes you will understand the opponent's intention. Then your heart (mind) will naturally and clearly react to the opponent's strategy. The eyes and the heart cannot be separated. They act like one. Only then can the body follow the heart's intention automatically and naturally without confusion.

9. Thesis of Stepping (Bu Fa Lun) 九 · 步法論

When the five sensing organs and hundred skeletonbones decide to move, in fact, they are transported by the stepping. The stepping is the foundation of the entire body and the governing key to movement. Therefore, engaging in battle and matching the opponent relies on the body, (but) actually the main support of this is nothing but stepping. (Although) the changes which correspond to the situation and opportunity are in the hands, however, that which enables the hands to switch and move around is also in the stepping. Advancing, retreating, turning around, and beware of the sides, if not for the stepping, how could (you) catch the opportunity to stimulate (the Qi) and also to raise, extend, and withdraw. If not for the stepping, how could (you) demonstrate the marvellous variations? What is called the tricky keys are in the eyes, the variations are (generated) in the heart. Then it is possible to turn around and change angles, thousand variations and ten thousand derivations which prevent (you) from being forced into an urgent (situation); if not from the actions of stepping, how could it be done? (However, all of these) goals cannot be reached by force.

今夫五官百骸，主於動，而實運以步。步乃一身之根基，
運動之樞紐也。以故應戰對敵，皆本諸身，而實所以為
身之砥柱者，莫非步。隨機應變在於手，而所以為手之
轉移者，亦在步。進退反側，非步何以作鼓盪之機，抑
揚伸縮，非步何以示變化之妙。所謂機關者在眼，變化
者在心。而所以轉灣抹角，千變萬化，而不至於窘迫者，
何莫非步之司命歟。而要非勉強以致之也。

It is the stepping which gives your strategy life and creates the hundreds of variations. It is also the stepping which allows you to react naturally to an attack and avoid or escape from dangerous situations. Although stepping is so important, all of these achievements cannot be done in one day. It will take a lot of practice and accumulated experience before you are able to reach this goal without forcing it. If you can only achieve these variations by force, then your attention is on the forcing, and your reactions will not be natural and automatic, and your stepping will not be effectively coordinated with your strategy.

The movements originate from no heart (i.e., no intention) and the excitement is generated from no feeling. When the body wishes to move, the stepping will also move around (automatically). When the hands are going to move, (you have) already stepped to the (opponent's) urgent position. This happens (naturally) without expectation, progresses without being pushed. Isn't this what is called the top wishes to move the bottom naturally follows? Furthermore, stepping is divided into front (leg) and rear (leg), the one with definite positions (i.e., the front leg) is stepping, also the one without definite positions (i.e., the rear leg) is also stepping. Such as the front leg steps forward, the rear leg will follow. The front and the rear all have a definite position. (However), if the earlier stepping (leg) steps later, and the later stepping (leg) steps first, also if the earlier stepping (leg) is used as the first stepping (leg) for the later, or the later stepping (leg) is used as the following stepping (leg) for the first, then the earlier and the later stepping (legs) will naturally not have definite positions. In all, when (we) talk about the situation of the fist (i.e., style), the important point should be considered to be stepping. Lively or not is also decided by stepping. Agile or not also depends on stepping. How great are the applications of stepping!

動作出於無心，鼓舞出於不覺，身欲動而步亦為之周旋，
手將動而步亦早為之催逼，不期然而然，莫之驅而驅。
所謂上欲動而下自隨之者，其斯之謂歟。且步分前後，
有定位者，步也；然而無定位者，亦為步。如前步進焉，
後步隨焉，前後自有定位。若以前步作後，後步作前，
更以前步作後之前步，後步作前之後步，則前後亦自然
無定位矣。總之拳以論勢，而握要者為步，活與不活，
亦在於步，靈與不靈，亦在於步，步之為用大矣哉。

Your strategy is from the heart, but your movements must be from your natural reactions. When a situation arises, everything happens very fast and you have no time to think. If you have not acquired natural, fast, and accurate reactions through your training, you have already lost the battle. In order to acquire this automatic fighting strategy you must train until every single part of your body is involved in every movement you make. Then, every tiny part of your body will be involved in the fighting. This means that when one part of your body moves, no part doesn't move, and if one part is calm, all parts are calm. Only then will your stepping and techniques be natural and effective. When you are at this stage, then there are no set rules.

Although your heart (emotional mind) normally determines your actions, you have to train until you can act automatically, without getting emotionally involved. In the same way, you have to raise your spirit without getting excited, because this would keep you from responding accurately.

The fist (i.e., this style) is named Xin-Yi (heart-mind). In Xin-Yi, the Yi (intention) originates from the Xin (heart) and the fists are emitted according to the Yi. (You) must know yourself and the opponent, following the opportunity and responding with variations. (When) the Qi in the heart is emitted, the four limbs all move. (When) the feet are raised, they are grounded. (When) the knees are lifted, they have number (i.e., specific techniques). (When) turning, there are positions. Combine with the shoulders and coordinate with the hips, three tips are matching, and the Xin, Yi, and Qi internal three are (also) combined. The fist is combined with the feet, the elbows are combined with the knees, and the shoulders are combined with the hips, external three are combined. The palm centers, the sole centers, and the Xin, three centers and one Qi are mutually combined. (When it is) far, the hands are not emitted. (When) the fists are used to strike within five feet and beyond three feet, (it does) not matter (whether moving) forward, retreating, moving to the left or to the right, every step corresponds with each fist (strike). The rule is (it is) marvellous if (it) is able to reach the opponent and (he) cannot see your shape.

捶名心意；心意者，意自心生，拳隨意發，總要知己知
人，隨機應變。心氣一發，四肢皆動，足起有地，膝起
有數，動轉有位，合膊望胯，三尖對照，心意氣內三相
合。拳與足合，肘與膝合，肩與胯合，外三相合。手心，
足心，本心，三心一氣相合。遠不發手，捶打五尺以內，
三尺以外，不論前後左右，一步一捶，發手以得人為準，
以不見形為妙。

Xingyiquan is sometimes called Xin Yi Quan (心意拳) because the heart (emotional mind) plays such an important role. Once the Xin is generated, the Yi takes over to provide clear judgement. Finally, the strategy is decided and the techniques are applied. The Xin and Yi are the masters of the fight, and once a decision has been made, action follows immediately. Normally, when the Xin is activated, the Qi in your entire body is stimulated for action. That is why it is said that when the Qi in the heart is emitted, the four limbs all move. The entire body moves as a unit, and the feet are always rooted. In addition, the three tips (tips of the nose, hands, and feet) must line up, the three internal combination (Xin, Yi, and Qi) and the three external combination (hands-feet, elbows-knees, and shoulders-hips) must also be established. Furthermore, in order to become a coherent unit in a fight, you must also combine the internal and external. All of these are the requirements of Xingyiquan.

When you are in the middle range, every time you step you should strike the opponent, and every time you strike the opponent you should step. When you act, do not express your intention in your face or reveal it in your posture. Then your opponent will not be able to figure out what you are going to do.

When the hands are emitted, (they are) fast like the wind and the arrow. (When shouting), the sound is like thunder. Appear and disappear like a rabbit. It is like a lively bird entering the woods. Encountering an enemy, (you are) like an giant cannon whose power can destroy a (thick) wall like a thin one. The eyes are sharp and the hands are fast. When you jump forward, it is straight forward for swallowing. Before exchanging hands, the Qi is already forward. Once the hands have entered (i.e., the fight has started), the agile movements are most marvellous. (When you) see an opening, do not strike. (When you) see the Heng, then strike. (When you) see the opening, do not stand firm. (When you) see the Heng, then stand firm. Top, middle, and bottom, hold the Qi steady. The body, feet, and hands are all following orders. They are not raised because of the opening and they do not fall because of the opening. The wisdom and skillful tricks all depend on the aliveness, ability to go, ability to fit in, ability to be soft, and ability to be hard, ability to advance, and ability to retreat, (when) not moving, steady as a mountain, as difficult to figure out as Yin and Yang, unlimited like the heavens and the earth, and full like a huge granary. (Your understanding) is extensive and (knowledge is) abundant as the four seas. (You are) bright and shinning like the three lights. Inspect the opportunity of the opponent's attack and determine the advantages and disadvantages. There are advanced techniques where (you are) calm and wait for the movement. There are borrowing techniques where (you) move to deal with the (opponent's) calmness. The borrowing techniques are easy and the advanced techniques are hard. The advanced techniques should still be considered first.

發手快似風，箭響如雷鳴，出沒如兔，亦如生鳥之投林。
應敵似巨炮推薄壁之勢，眼明手快，踴躍直吞，未曾交
手，一氣當先，既入其手，靈動為妙。見孔不打，見橫
打，見孔不立，見橫立，上中下總氣把定。身足手規矩
繩束，既不望空起，亦不望空落。精明靈巧，全在於活，
能去能就，能柔能剛，能進能退，不動如山岳，難知如
陰陽，無窮如天地，充實如太倉，浩渺如四海，炫曜如
三光。察來勢之機會，揣敵人之短長。靜以待動有上法，
動以處靜有借法。借法容易上法難，還是上法最為先。

This section exposes the deeper secrets of fighting. The depth of your fighting experience will determine how much you really comprehend of the profound contents of this paragraph.

The first few sentences state again the feeling and the appearance of the actions. The hands move like the wind or an arrow, the sound is loud like thunder, the techniques are applied as swiftly as a rabbit, the movements are mysterious and hard to see as a tiny bird flying through the trees, the power is like an cannon, the eyes are like an eagle's, and when you jump forward it is like a tiger pouncing on a lamb. All of these are done through the Qi, which itself is led by the Yi. Once you have engaged in a fight, the agility is the marvellous key to winning.

The second few sentences of this section discuss strategy. When you see an opening in the opponent's posture, you should not automatically attack, because it could be a trap. You are usually aware of when your own posture has a gap or opening, and sometimes use it to entice the opponent into attacking in a predictable way that you are prepared to counter. However, when you see that you have a chance to enwrap the opponent's hands or force them to the side ("when you see the Heng"), then you may attack. When you force or lead the opponent's limbs away, his mind is on defending against your actions, and this creates an opening for your attack. When you see the opening, do not be so determined to attack that you become inflexible, because your opponent may have exposed himself on purpose, and is prepared for your attack. Instead, you should move around and change the angle and position. This will force the opponent to change his strategy and set a new trap. While he is changing, you have an opportunity to attack. However, if you are able to apply Heng to enwrap the opponent's attack to the side, then you should stand firm in order to build up the root for a powerful strike.

All of your strategy and reactions should not be based on apparent openings in the opponent's posture. You should be alert and apply your wisdom skillfully to the actual situation. Then your techniques can be soft or hard, and you can move forward or backward according to the situation. Your thinking and movements should be changeable like Yin and Yang so that your opponent cannot figure out what you intend to do.

You should also continue to increase your knowledge and experience until they are as abundant as the oceans. Your spirit should be as bright as the three lights (San

Guang, 三光), which are the sun, the moon, and the stars, so that you can clearly see the advantageous and disadvantageous situations.

The last few sentences of this section talk about techniques. The best and most advanced technique is to keep yourself very calm and alert, and wait patiently for the opponent's first move. There is a martial arts proverb that says: "When the enemy does not move, I do not move. When the enemy moves slightly, then I move first." When the opponent does not move, his whole heart (attention) is on preparing for your attack. If you attack at this time, you will not be successful. Therefore, you should keep calm and alert with him. However, once he starts to move just slightly, his Yi is revealed and he is concentrating on his new intention. At this time, his mind is not on defending. If you can catch this timing and move fast, you may interrupt his intention and confuse him. When this happens, you have a good chance to succeed. If you are interested in more on fighting strategy, please refer to the book, *Tai Chi Chuan, Martial Applications*, by Dr. Yang.

However, if your opponent remains calm for a long time, you may want to do something to make him move first. Then you have to borrow a technique. This means that you temporarily "borrow" a technique to use it as a fake—it is not your actual attack. Such techniques cause the opponent to move and break down his concentration on his defense. Naturally, when you use these fakes you must be very alert for his reaction. The text reminds you that the best technique is to wait until your opponent moves first. If you have to borrow a faking technique, then your attention will be on your offensive strategy and your defense will be weak for a moment. Therefore, borrowing techniques are not as good as waiting techniques.

Those who are exchanging bravery (i.e., fighting) should not think about mistakes (already made). Those who think about the mistakes find it hard to move even an inch step. (The movement) rises like a penetrating arrow and falls like the wind. (When) the hands grasp the hands, attack forward. Every movement automatically combines secretly. Speedy like lighting in the sky and beware of the two sides, left and right. Turning to the rear is just like a tiger searching the mountain. (When) chop and strike are used, (they are) intrepid and undefeatable. Chop the endings (i.e., limbs) and attack the face, aiming for the Zhongtang. (When) thrusting upward and downward, it is like a tiger, also like an eagle swooping downward to a chicken coop. Do not be hurried in turning over the rivers and reversing the ocean. A single phoenix who dares to fly toward the sun can be said to be brave. (When) the clouds are covering the heavens and the moon, the heavens and the earth interact (i.e., there is a storm); when martial arts are competed the winner and the loser can be seen.

交勇者，不可思誤，思誤者，寸步難行。起如箭鑽落如風，手樓手分向前攻。舉動暗中自合，疾如閃電在天。兩邊攔防左右，反背如虎搜山。斬捶勇猛不可當，斬梢迎面取中堂。搶上搶下勢如虎，好似鷹鶻下雞場。翻江倒海不須忙，單鳳朝陽才為強。雲背日月天地交，武藝相爭見短長。

While fighting, you should not be thinking about errors you have made. If you are doing this, you are not concentrating on the fight, and so your stepping and use of techniques will be stagnant. The text then goes on to describe how the Yi should be manifested in the movements. Zhongtang (中堂) means the center of the face.

When stepping, an inch apart and step a foot. Chop forward to the face and step the right leg and advance with left steps, following this method to move forward. (When) approaching the opponent (to attack), advance your body. (When) the body and the hands arrive together, then (the techniques) can be real. Within the emitting, how do (we) understand the secret application? When the meaning has been explained, its marvelousness can seem to be supernatural. When a bird of prey enters the woods, it must not catch its wings. (When) an eagle is seizing a small bird, its postures are balanced in four directions. To win the victory, the four extremities must be gathered neatly. First, (you) still need the hand to protect the heart. Plan the strategies and apply them skillfully, a spirit of thunder and a venomous heart is the best policy. (Then) the hands and the eyes are able to defeat the opponent.

步路寸開把尺，劈面就去。上右腿，進左步，此法前行。進人要進身，身手齊到是為真。發中有絕何從用，解明其意妙如神。鷂子鑽林莫著翅，鷹捉小鳥勢四平。取勝四梢要聚齊，第一還要手護心。計謀施運化，霹靂走精神。心毒稱上策，手眼方勝人。

When you step forward, avoid a wide stance and keep your feet only an inch or so apart. When you step, only step about a foot each time. This way you will always maintain a firm stance and an effective defensive posture. The two legs should take turns advancing. When you advance, the body must also move together with the stepping and occupy the opponent's center door (Zhong Men, 中門). When you attack, your stepping, body, and hands must all arrive at the same time in order to be effective ("real"). This is the secret of emitting. How can a person really catch this secret if it is not explained to him and he is able to comprehend the real meaning behind it?

When you attack, you must avoid having your technique interrupted, like a bird flying into the woods and catching its wing on a branch. You must also be calm, firm, and balanced in all directions like an eagle catching a bird. In addition to good strategy and good protection, you must also have a sharp and mean look and a raised spirit, then you will be able to win.

What is dodging? What is advancing? To advance is to dodge and to dodge is to advance. Do not look for the distant answer. What is called a strike? What is called beware? To beware is to strike and to strike is to beware. The hands are just simply emitted. The heart is like gun powder and the fist is like a cannon ball. When the trigger is moved, it is hard for the bird to fly (away). The body is like a bow and bowstring and the hands are like the arrows. When the string is aimed at the bird, the marvelous results will be seen. When the hands move, like lightning; lightning is so fast that there is not enough time to close the eyes. The striking is like thunder and it is so fast that (you) do not have time to cover your ears. The five paths are actually the five entrances. Nobody protects them but yourself. When the left hand passes the cheek (to block), the right hand will go (to attack). When the right cheek's hand is going, the left cheek's hand is coming. The two hands are bound (into) fists (i.e., held tight) and released to the (opponent's) face. The doors of the five gates are tightly closed. The fists are emitted from the heart and fall onto the (opponent's) nose. The feet are (grown) from underneath the ground. When a foot is raised fast, the heart Fire is flaming. The Five Phases are Metal, Wood, Water, Fire, and Earth. The Fire is flaming upward and the Water is flowing downward. (If) I have (the coordination of) the heart, liver, spleen, lungs, and kidneys, then the Five Phases can mutually cooperate without mistake.

何謂閃？何謂進？進即閃，閃即進，不必遠求。何謂打？
何謂顧？顧即打，打即顧，發手便是。心如火藥拳如子，
靈機一動鳥難飛；身似弓弦手似箭，弦向鳥落見神奇。
起手如閃電，閃電不及合眸；打人如迅雷，迅雷不及掩
耳。五道本是五道關，無人把守自遮攔。左腮手過來，
右腮手去。右腮手過去，左腮手來。兩手束拳迎面出，
五關之門關得嚴。拳從內心發，向鼻尖落。足從地下起，
足起快時心火作。五行金木水火土，火炎上而水就下。
我有心肝脾肺腎，五行相推無錯誤。

In a fight, a dodge can be used as an advance and an advance can be used as a dodge. A strike can be a defense and a defense can be an attack. You should not be bothered with trying to distinguish all of these. Simply react naturally and automatically.

It is not clear what the five paths (Wu Dao, 五道) are that the document refers to. Since the five paths are considered to be the five gates which the opponent is able to enter, they may be the face, chest, abdomen, groin, and shin, which are the five common zones for an attack. However, it may imply the five directions which the enemy may enter, the front, rear, left, right, and center.

---

10. Thesis of Fighting (Jiao Shou Lun) 十 · 交手論

Grab the right, enter the left. Grab the left, enter the right. When stepping forward, the heels touch the ground first. The tip of the foot uses the toes to grab the ground. The stepping must be steady and the body must be solemn. The strike must be firm, solid, and have Li from the bones. While going (i.e., attacking), the hands are relaxed and when they reach the opponent they become fists. When fists are used, curl (the fingers) in tightly. When you grab, the grabbing must have Qi. From the top to the bottom, the Qi must be uniform. Exiting (i.e., attacking) and entering (i.e., withdrawing) use the heart as master. The eyes, hands, and feet then follow. Do not be greedy and do not be deficient. The elbows should fall into the cave of the elbows (i.e., their prescribed position) and the hands should fall into the hands' cave. The right leg moves first and the tip of the shoulder (i.e., hands) moves forward. This is (the secret of) exchanging steps.

占右進左，占左進右。發步時足跟先著地，足尖以十趾
抓地。步要穩當，身要莊重。捶要沉實而有骨力。去是
撒手，著人成拳。用拳要捲緊，用把把有氣。上下氣要
均停，出入以心為主宰。眼手足隨之去，不貪不歉，不
即不離，肘落肘窩，手落手窩。右足當先，膊尖向前，
此是換步。

When you attack, the two hands coordinate with each other and the feet are rooted. The stepping is steady and the body is solid and stable ("solemn"). When you strike, the Qi comes from deep in the bones (i.e., the marrow). The key to leading the Qi to the fist when striking is to relax in the beginning of the punch so that the Qi can be led to the fist by the Yi smoothly and without stagnation. Right before this fist arrives at the opponent's body, the fist should be tightened up firmly so that the forward power is firmly supported by the middle and the root section. This also keeps the fist from being injured.

Qi is also important in grabbing because it makes the grab powerful and irresistible. In all things, the heart is always the master. When using a technique, beware of trying too hard or attempting too much, but also avoid holding back and slighting the techniques. Your posture should always be correct, and all of the key parts of your body, such as the fists and elbows, should be positioned correctly This seals the vital areas of your body from attack.

The fist is emitted from the heart, and the hand is urged by the body. The hand is grabbing with the heart and the heart is grabbing with the hand. (When) the man moves and steps forward, every step and every fist, one branch moves, hundreds of branches all follow. There is a secret in emitting Jin, when one (hand) is grabbing, the entire body is all grabbing, when one is extending, the entire body is all extending. Extending must extend enough to enter, the grabbing must grab to the root. Like wrapping the cannon, (must) wrap tightly, and restrained with Li. It does not matter whether lift striking, press striking, ward off striking, rotating striking, chopping striking, thrusting striking, drilling striking, elbow striking, shoulder striking, palm striking, head striking, forward step striking, backward step striking, smooth step striking, sideways step striking, and front, rear, left, right, top, and bottom, all hundreds of striking methods, all must mutually follow (each other). (When) releasing hands (i.e., attacking), first occupy the front door. This is called cunning.

拳從心發，以身力催手，手以心把，心以手把，進人進
步，一步一捶，一支動，百支俱隨。發中有絕，一握渾
身皆握，一伸渾身皆伸。伸要伸得進，握要握得根。如
捲炮，捲得緊，弸得有力。不拘提打、按打、烘打、旋
打、斬打、沖打、錛打、肘打、膊打、胯掌打、頭打、
進步打、退步打、順步打、橫步打、以及前後左右上下
百般打法，皆要一齊相隨。出手先占正門，此之謂巧。

A strike originates from the heart, and the hand is urged forward by the body. When you grab, your mind and the actual grabbing cannot be separated. The mind and the action must be united. In every movement, when one part moves, the entire body moves. The secret of emitting Jin is that the entire body acts as a unit. When you strike, the strike must be far enough to reach the opponent and when you grab, you must grab right down to the opponent's root. In all extending and grabbing techniques, your arms should feel like wrapped cannon, and the muscles should be strongly tensed. Muzzle loading cannon were sometimes wrapped with wire to make them stronger. This way they could be loaded with more powder so that they could shoot farther. Your arms should have these two balancing forces in them. They should be continually extending and expanding, but at the same time they should be held in and contained. Regardless of which technique you use, you must follow one simple rule: the entire body must act as a unit. The trick to seizing the advantage is to occupy the opponent's front door as much as possible. This puts him into a defensive and urgent position.

> *The bone sections must be matched, (if) not matched, no Li. The hand grabbing must be agile, (if) not agile, then changes can occur. The emitting hand must be fast, (if) not fast, then too late. The rising hand must be alive, (if) not alive, then not fast. Striking must have follow-up, (if) no follow-up, then not effective. The scheming heart must be venomous, (if) not venomous, then not accurate. Feet and hands must be alive, (if) not alive, then (they) carry danger. The scheming heart must be refined, (if) not refined, then it will be fooled. (When) attacking, must be brave and fierce like an eagle's stoop. (Be) calm externally and audacious, and use the opportunity skillfully. Must not be afraid, hesitant, and suspicious (i.e., worried). The heart is small (i.e. refined) and the bladder is big (i.e., brave). The face looks nice, the mind is venomous. Be calm like a scholar and move like the thunder striking.*

> 骨節要對，不對則無力。手把要靈，不靈則生變。發手
> 要快，不快則遲誤。舉手要活，不活則不快。打手要跟，
> 不跟則不濟。存心要毒，不毒則不準。腳手要活，不活
> 則擔險。存心要精，不精則受愚。發作要鷹捉勇猛，外
> 靜膽大，機要熟運，切勿畏懼遲疑，心小膽大，面善心
> 惡，靜似書生，動如雷發。

The three sections must be coordinated with each other, otherwise they will not be able to support each other and the Li will be weak. Grabbing must be fast and agile so that the opponent has no chance to change his strategy. When you attack, you must be like an eagle swooping down to attack its prey (stooping). In addition, the strikes must be fast, the mind must be clear and sharp, techniques must be alive, etc. All of these ideas are repeated from other well-known documents.

> *The opponent's approaching posture must also be carefully inspected, such as the feet's kicks, the head's bump, the fist's strikes and the shoulder's action, narrowing the body to advance, relying on the body to raise and emit, walking diagonally and exchanging stepping, intercepting strikes and retreating the body, and lifting and extending the leg for emitting (i.e., kicking). (When) you are wary of (the opponent's) feet to the east, must prevent (being) killed from the west. (When) the top is void, the bottom must be solid. The tricks (are so many that)*

the fingers are not enough for bending (i.e., counting). The clever tricks and opportunities must be figured out by yourself. The fast hand strikes the slow hand. The traditional sayings should not be ignored. (They) indeed have their knowledgeable opinion.

人之來勢，亦當審察。腳踢頭撞，拳打膊作。窄身進步，
仗身起發。斜行換步，攔打倒身，抬腿伸發。腳指東顧，
須防西殺。上虛下必實著，詭計指不勝屈。靈機自揣摩，
手急打手慢。俗言不可輕，的確有識見。

In a fight, you must not only consider your own attack, you must also concern yourself with how your opponent can attack you. Only then will you realize the opponent's intention, strategy, and techniques. All of this comes from careful inspection and clear judgement. It is nothing else but wise thinking and the accumulation of experience over a long period of training.

(When) rising, expect falling. (When) falling, expect rising. The rising and falling mutually follow each other. (The techniques which) the body and the hands all arrive at the same time are the real (techniques). The thighs form a scissors and (the hands) chop toward the (opponent's) eyebrows (i.e., face). In addition, turning around is like a tiger searching the mountain. The hands rise like lighting and fall like the speedy thunder, (like) the wind blowing the rain, the eagle seizing the swallow, the sparrow hawk entering the woods, and the lion catching a rabbit. When the hands are raised, the three centers match each other. (When) not moving, like a scholar and (when you) move, like a dragon and a tiger. (If) too far, the hands should not be emitted for striking. Two hands protect the sides of the heart. (When) an attack is from the right, (I) intercept with the right (hand) and (when) an attack is from the left, (I) intercept with the left. This is a short cut in intercepting. If too far, then (I) move forward with my hand and when it is close, (then) add the elbow (strike). If it is far, then use the leg to kick and if it is close, (then) add the knee (strike). Far or close must be known properly. The fist's strike and the foot's kick (come) from the head to the postures; inspecting the opponent can cause you to think of advancing. (If) there is an Yi, do not have shape (i.e., external appearance). (If) there is a shape, then (you) will not win.

起望落，落望起，起落覆相隨，身手齊到是為真。剪子
股，望眉斬，加上反背，如虎搜山。起手如閃電，打下
如迅雷，雨行風，鷹捉燕，鷂鑽林，獅搏兔。起手時三
心相對，不動如書生，動之如龍虎。遠不發手打，雙手
護心旁。右來右迎，左來左迎，此為捷取。遠了便上手，
近了便加肘。遠了便腳踢，近了便加膝。遠近宜知。拳
打足踢，頭至把勢，審人能叫一思進。有意莫帶形，帶
形必不贏。

In a fight, when your opponent is rising you should expect him to fall, and when he is falling you should expect him to rise. The same theory can apply to you. When you rise, you are already getting ready to fall. When you fall, your mind has already prepared to rise. This is simply because rising and falling are a common strategy for confusing the opponent and preventing him from protecting his upper and lower body at the same time.

The legs should be held close together like a pair of scissors. This protects the groin and keeps the stance stable. The three centers are the top of the head directing downward, the bottoms of the feet directing upward, and the center where the Qi is directed inward from the hands.

The last two sentences mean that when your Yi has decided to do something, you should conceal your intentions so that your opponent will not be able to determine what you are going to do.

> *The method of defeating the opponent: inspect and be aware of the shape of the ground. (When) a fist is in an advantageous position, the hands must be speedy. The feet must be light (i.e., agile) and when the postures are moving, they are like a cat's walk. The heart (i.e., mind) must be neutral and centered, the eyes are gathering essence (i.e., concentrated), (when) the hands and feet all arrive, (I) must win. If the hands arrive but the feet are not arriving, then (I) cannot obtain the marvellous trick. (If) the hands arrive and the feet also arrive, (then) striking the opponent is just like pulling up grass (i.e., easy). The top strikes the throat and the bottom strikes the groin. The left or the right flank remains in the center. It is not far to strike ten feet away. (When) it is close, it can be within only an inch.*

捷取人法，審顧地形，拳打上風，手要急，足要輕，把
勢走動如貓行。心要正，目聚精，手足齊到定要贏。若
是手到步不到，打人不得妙。手到步也到，打人如拔草。
上打咽喉下打陰，左右兩脅在中心。前打一丈不為遠，
近者只在一寸間。

When you are about to get involved in a fight, first you must know the ground, such as where it is high and where it is low, where it is hard and where it is soft, which direction faces the sun and the wind, where it is slippery and where it is firm. Only then can you skillfully take advantage of the surroundings and use them in your fight. For example, avoid facing the sun and wind, and beware of being forced into disadvantageous situations. Naturally, you would like to put your opponent into the disadvantageous position. Once you have the opportunity to attack, you must use speed, otherwise your chance will soon pass.

When you fight, your body should be turned to the corner so that the front of your body is not so exposed to the opponent. The elbows are kept down to protect your center. This "triangular" position enables you to reach far yet not expose too much of your body. When you move, the stepping must be agile and fast, the mind centered and not distracted, the eyes concentrated, and the entire body acting as one unit. I can strike the top and the bottom as I wish while still protecting the center of my body. If I can achieve these requirements, then even if the opponent is ten feet away, it is not too far for me to attack, and if the opponent is even only an inch away, I still have enough skill to defeat him.

When the body moves, (it is) like a wall collapsing. When the feet are falling (to the ground), (it is) like a tree is growing roots. When the hands are rising, (it is) like a fired cannonball, thrusting straight forward. The body should be like a living snake, when the head is attacked, the tail will respond, when the tail is attacked, the head will respond, and when the middle sections is attacked, the head and the tail both respond. When striking forward, must be aware of the rear. Knowing (how to move) forward, you should also know (how to move) backward. The heart moves like a horse, the shoulders move with the speed of wind. When training it seems there is someone in front of you and when you are exchanging the hands (i.e., fighting), even though there is an opponent, it is like fighting nobody. When the front hand rises, the rear hand urges closely. When the front leg rises, the rear leg follows closely. (Though) there are hands in front of you, do not see the hands and (though) there are elbows in front of (your) chest, (you) do not see the elbows.

身動時如崩牆倒，腳落時如樹栽根。手起如炮直沖，身
要如活蛇，擊首則尾應，擊尾則首應，擊中節而首尾皆
相應。打前要顧後，知進須知退。心動快似馬，臂動速
如風。操演時面前如有人，交手時有人如無人。起前手，
後手緊催，起前腳，後腳緊跟。面前有手不見手，胸前
有肘不見肘。

When your body starts to act, it can be as powerful as a collapsing wall. Once your feet contact the ground, they are immediately rooted. When you strike, your hand is as fast as a cannonball.

In addition, you must connect your head, middle, and end sections and make them act as one. When any section is attacked, the other two will respond naturally. You must also beware of the four directions, the front, the rear, and the two sides. When the heart starts to act (when you decide to act), it is like a running horse: it moves quickly but the mind is clear. In Chinese Qigong the monkey is used to represent the emotional mind: excited, unsteady, and running around without a firm plan. The horse, on the other hand, represents the wisdom mind, which is calm and steady, and is able to move rapidly with assurance.

When you train, visualize an opponent in front of you. However, when you are actually fighting with someone, if you have trained properly you will have developed enough skill and power that it will seem like the opponent isn't even there, and you will cut right through him. In Qigong it is said: the real regulating is no regulating. This means that when your mind still has to pay attention and conduct the act, then you are regulating the act. However, once you have mastered the act, you do not need to put your mind wholly on it, and can act automatically and naturally. This is the regulating without regulating. It is just like when you are learning how to drive, your mind is on the driving. However, after you have driven for many years, all of the reactions have become natural, and you do not have to pay attention to all the details.

If (you) see an opening, do not strike, and if (you) see the opening, do not advance. The fist should not strike the false rising and also not strike the false lowering. (When) the hands rise, the feet must fall. When the feet fall, the hands must rise. The heart must move first and the Yi must defeat the opponent. The body will attack the opponent (first) and the stepping must be better than the opponent's. The front leg is like crossing (i.e., like a snake) and the rear leg is like sticking. The head must stick up and the chest must be exposed (i.e., thrust out). The waist must grow and rise, and the Dan Tian must transport the Qi (smoothly). From the top to the feet, the one Qi must thread through. (If) afraid in the battle and the heart is cold, (then) surely not able to win. (If) unable to inspect the talking and view the color (of the face), surely not able to prevent the opponent's (intention) and surely not able to move first. (He who) moves first is the master, and (he who) moves second is the follower. Be able to think only of advancing and do not keep thinking of retreating.

如見空不打，見空不上。拳不打空起，亦不打空落。手起足要落，足落手要起。心要占先，意要勝人，身要攻人，步要過人，前腿似翘，後腿似忝，手要仰起，胸要現起，腰要長起，丹田要運氣。自頂至足，要一氣相貫，膽戰心寒，必不能取勝，未能察言觀色者，必不能防人，必不能先動。先動為師，後動為弟，能叫一思進，莫叫一思退。

When you see an opening while your opponent's mind is calm and his postures are ordered, then this opening can be a trap, therefore do not attack. Your opponent may try to trick you by raising or lowering his body in order to lure you into a trap. However, you should understand that if the opponent's hands are rising, his legs must be rooting, and he will not be able to kick. Similarly, when he is kicking his root is weak, and his hands will not be in a good position to emit Jin. If you can comprehend these secrets, then you will be able to find the right opportunity for your attack.

The key to winning is staying alert and responding earlier than the opponent. In addition, your Yi must be able to judge the situation clearly, quickly, and make a firm decision on what to do. Only then will your body be able to act first, and your stepping be agile and effective.

When your front leg steps, it moves in curves like a snake so that it can get into the best position. However, when you use your front leg to enter the opponent's empty door, the rear leg must remain firm and rooted, and then immediately follow the front leg. The head should be held up, and the chest lifted, so that your spirit can be raised to a high level. Your waist must be flexible and agile. In order to manifest your fighting power, the Qi must be threaded through your entire body so that it functions as a unit.

Next, in order to win a battle, you must not be afraid, because this disturbs your mind and prevents you from thinking wisely or even observing the opponent's intentions. If this happens, you will always be on the defensive, and you will be certain to lose.

The three sections must be clear, the three tips must match, and the four extremities must be gathered. Understanding the three centers will increase by one more power, comprehending the three sections will add one more technique, understanding the four extremities will increase one essence, understanding the Five Phases will increase the one Qi. Understanding the three sections, not greedy and not deficient, rise, fall, advance, and retreat will have more variations. Three rounds and nine turns are one posture (i.e., in each posture). All must be mastered by the one heart. Using the two Qis (i.e., inhalation and exhalation) to govern the Five Phases, practice all the time, do not be delayed morning and evening. Crossing the legs (for meditation) and striking (for form practice) must often be forced. After the Gong (i.e., Gongfu: energy and time) has passed, it will be natural. This is sincere language and not empty talk.

三節要停，三尖要照，四梢要齊。明了三心多一方，明了三節多一方，明了四梢多一精，明了五行多一氣。明了三節，不貪不歉，起落進退多變，三回九轉是一勢，總要一心為主宰。統乎五行，運乎二氣，時時操演，勿誤朝夕。盤打時而勉強，工用久而自然。誠哉是言，豈虛語哉。

Finally, this article reviews some of the key points of the training. You must understand the three sections clearly, because this enables you to use your body skillfully and increases the number of variations of the techniques that you can perform. The three tips (nose, fingers, and toes) must match. This keeps your posture firm and rooted, and makes it possible for you to increase your power. The three centers were mentioned earlier. They are the center of the head directed downward, the centers of the feet pointing upward, and the centers of the hands aiming inward. The Qi must be able to reach the four extremities (tongue, hair, teeth, and nails) so that your Qi will be strong. However, in order to have abundant Qi, you must know how to increase the efficiency of the Essence-Qi conversion. With the knowledge of the Five Phases (Five Internal Organs), the Qi can be threaded together and become one.

It does not matter where or how you fight, these key requirements remain the same. Inhalation and exhalation are the keys to governing the Qi in the Five Organs. Practice hard and ceaselessly, and some day you will find that all of these requirements have become a part of you. Once this happens, you will surely be a proficient fighter.

Glossary of Chinese Terms

An Shen Pao 安身炮

Secure Body Strike. Name of a two-person matching set in Xingyiquan. This matching set is designed for beginners to practice the skills of Five Fists (Wu Quan, 五拳).

Ba Duan Jin 八段錦

Eight Pieces of Brocade. One of the oldest medical Qigong set created by Marshal Yue, Fei during Chinese Southern Song Dynasty (1127-1280 A.D.).

Ba Shi Quan 八式拳

Eight Postures Sequence. Name of a Xingyiquan barehand sequence.

Bagua 八卦

Literally: Eight Divinations. Also called the Eight Trigrams. In Chinese philosophy, the eight basic variations; shown in the Yi Jing (易經) as groups of single and broken lines.

Baguazhang 八卦掌

Literally: Bagua Palm. A style of Chinese internal martial arts which was created based on the theory of the Bagua (i.e., Eight Trigrams) theory.

Bai He 白鶴

White Crane. A well known southern Chinese martial style which originated in the Shaolin Temple (少林寺).

Bao 抱

Bao be translated as embrace, hold together, stick together, enfold, harbor, or cherish. One of the basic techniques in Xingyiquan training.

Beng Quan 弸拳

One of the Five Fists (Wu Quan, 五拳) in Xingyiquan.

Cai 踩

To step.

Ce 側

Sides. It means to beware of the sides in Xingyiquan.

Chang Chuan (Changquan) 長拳

Chang means long, and Chuan means fist, style, or sequence. A style of Northern Chinese Gongfu (功夫) which specializes in kicking and long range fighting. Chang Chuan has also been used to refer to Taijiquan.

Chen Jia Gou 陳家溝

Chen's Village. A famous village located at Zheng Zhou, Henan Province, China (河南・鄭州), where the Chen family style of Taijiquan originated.

Cheng, Gin-Gsao (1911-1976 A.D.) 曾金灶

One of the authors, Dr. Yang's White Crane master.

Chengjiang (Co-24) 承漿

An acupuncture cavity located underneath the lips.

Chi (Qi) 氣

The general definition of Qi is: universal energy, including heat, light, and electromagnetic energy. A narrower definition of Qi refers to the energy circulating in human or animal bodies.

Chin Na (Qin Na) 擒拿

Literally, seize control. A type of Chinese Gongfu which emphasizes grabbing techniques to control the opponent's joints in conjunction with attacking certain acupuncture cavities. One of the main fighting categories in Chinese martial arts. These four categories are: kicking (Ti, 踢), striking (Da, 打), wrestling (Shuai, 摔), and controlling (Qin Na, 擒拿).

Chui 垂

Means to drop, fall, sink, or bow. One of the training key words in Xingyiquan.

Cun Bu 寸步

Literally: Inch Stepping. One of the advancing skills in stepping forward and backward.

Chuo Jiao 戳腳

Literally, "stamp foot." A Chinese martial style specializing in leg techniques.

Da Mo 達磨

The Indian Buddhist monk who is credited with creating the Yi Jin Jing (易筋經) and Xi Sui Jing (洗髓經) while at the Shaolin monastery. His last name was Chadili (剎地利), and he was also known as Bodhidarma. He was once the prince of a small tribe in southern India.

Da Peng Qigong 大鵬氣功

A style of Qigong which originated in Emei Mountain (峨嵋山).

Dan Tian 丹田

Literally: Elixir Field. Locations in the body which are able to store and generate

Qi (elixir) in the body. The Upper, Middle, and Lower Dan Tians are located respectively between the eyebrows (brain), at the lower section of stern (Jiuwei cavity, 鳩尾), and a few inches below the navel.

Dao 道
The way. The "natural" way of everything.

Di 低
Means low or falling. One of the fighting strategic actions in Xingyiquan.

Di 地
Earth.

Dian Xue An Mo 點穴按摩
Cavity Press Massage. One of the healing massages in Chinese medical practice.

Dihe (M-HN-19) 地閣
An acupuncture cavity which is located under Chengjiang cavity (承漿).

Ding 頂
Means to press. One of the fighting skills in Xingyiquan.

Du 毒
It has the meanings of poisonous, noxious, venomous, malicious, and spiteful in Chinese.

Du Mai 督脈
Governing Vessel. One of the Eight Extraordinary Vessels in Chinese medicine and Qigong.

Emei Mountain 峨嵋山
A mountain in Sichuan Province (四川省) where many martial styles originated.

Emei Wushu 峨嵋武術
Chinese martial arts created and developed in Emei Mountain.

Fan 反
Means to reverse or to turn around.

Fan 翻
Means to turn over.

Fei 飛
To fly.

Gansu 甘肅
A province of China.

Gao 高
Means high or rising. One of the strategic fighting actions in Xingyiquan.

Gongfu (Kung Fu) 功夫
Literally: energy-time. Any study, learning, or practice which requires a lot of patience, energy, and time to complete. Since practicing Chinese martial arts

requires a great deal of time and energy, Chinese martial arts are commonly called Gongfu.

Guai Zi Ma 拐子馬

Name of an ancient version of the tank. It was a chariot carrying armored men, drawn by three fully armored horses which were connected by a chain. Guai Zi Ma was a powerful weapons used by Jin race (金)(i.e., Mongolian) during Chinese Song Dynasty (960-1280 A.D.).

Guo 裹

To enwrap. One of the fighting skills in Xingyiquan.

Guoshu (Kuoshu) 國術

Literally: national techniques. Another name for Chinese martial arts. First used by President Chiang, Kai-Shek (蔣介石) in 1928 at the rounding of the Nanjing Central Guoshu Institute (南京中央國術館).

Haidi 海底

Means "sea bottom" which implies the tongue or the perineum area.

Han, Ching-Tang 韓慶堂

Dr. Yang, Jwing-Ming's Long Fist grandmaster.

Heng 横

Means sideways.

Heng Quan 横拳

Means sideway fist. One of the Five Fists (Wu Quan, 五拳) in Xingyiquan.

Hong Fan 洪範

The Great Plan. It is the title of one section of the *Book of History* (*Shi Ji*, 史記).

Hou Tian 後天

Post-Heaven. It means after birth.

Hou Tian Fa 後天法

Post Heaven Techniques. An internal style of martial Qigong which is believed to have been created around the sixth century.

Hu Kou 虎口

Tiger's Mouth, which is the martial arts term for the place between the thumb and the index finger.

Hua Mountain 華山

A sacred mountain in Shanxi Province (陝西省. One of the five great mountains in China. These five great mountains are: Tai Mountain (泰山)(east), Heng Mountain (衡山)(south), Hua Mountain (華山)(west), Heng Mountain (恆山)(north), and Song Mountain (嵩山)(center).

Huiyin (Co-1) 會陰

Literally: Meet Yin. An acupuncture cavity located at the perineum area.

Huo 火

Fire. One of the Five Phases.

Ji Bu 疾步

Urgent stepping. One of the strategic fighting actions in Xingyiquan.

Jiaji 夾脊

A Daoist term. Literally: Squeeze Spine. It is located between the shoulder blades. Jiaji is called Lingtai (Gv-10)(靈臺) in Chinese medicine.

Jin 金

Metal. One of the Five Phases.

Jin 進

Means to enter or to advance.

Jin 勁

A power in Chinese martial arts which is derived from muscles which have been energized by Qi to their maximum potential.

Jin Pai 金牌

An imperial order with the emperor's official golden seal.

Jin race 金人

Mongolian.

Jin, Shao-Feng 金紹峰

Dr. Yang, Jwing-Ming's White Crane grandmaster.

Jing 涇

A large river in Gansu Province (甘肅省) in China. This river flows into Shanxi Province (陝西省) where it joins with the Wei river (渭河).

Jing 精

Essence. The most refined part of anything.

Jing Zhong Bao Guo 精忠報國

It means to be loyal and pure to serve your country.

Jue 決

It means quick decision or thrusting. One of the strategic fighting actions in Xingyiquan.

Jue Ming 覺明

Literally: feel clear. It means to have a clear perception and understanding.

Jue Xiang 絕象

Means to stop imagination.

Kan 坎

A phase of the Eight Trigrams representing Water.

Kao, Tao 高濤

Dr. Yang, Jwing-Ming's first Taijiquan master.

Kong Men 空門

Literally "empty door." A Chinese martial arts term referring to an open or exposed area in a person's posture where the opponent can step in and attack a vital area.

Kou 扣

Means to arc or grab. One of the strategic fighting movements in Xingyiquan.

Kun 坤

One of the Eight Trigrams which represents the earth.

Laogong (P-8) 勞宮

An acupuncture cavity which is located at the center of the palms.

Kung Fu (Gongfu) 功夫

Literally: energy-time. Any study, learning, or practice which requires a lot of patience, energy, and time to complete. Since practicing Chinese martial arts requires a great deal of time and energy, Chinese martial arts are commonly called Gongfu.

Kuoshu (Guoshu) 國術

Literally: national techniques. Another name for Chinese martial arts. First used by President Chiang, Kai-Shek (蔣介石) in 1928 at the rounding of the Nanjing Central Guoshu Institute (南京中央國術館).

Li 力

The power which is generated from muscular strength.

Li 離

A phase of the Eight Trigrams representing Fire.

Li, Mao-Ching 李茂清

Dr. Yang, Jwing-Ming's Long Fist master.

Lian Jing Hua Qi 練精化氣

To refine the Essence and convert it into Qi.

Lian Qi 練氣

Means to train, to strengthen, and to refine the Qi.

Lian Qi Hua Shen 練氣化神

To refine the Qi to nourish the spirit. Leading Qi to the head to nourish the brain and spirit.

Lian Shen Fan Xu 練神返虛

To train the spirit to return to nothingness. An advanced stage of enlightenment and Buddhahood training in which the practitioner learns how to lead his spirit to separate from his physical body.

Liang, Shou-Yu 梁守渝

One of the authors of this book.

Liangong Shi Ba Fa Qigong 練功十八法氣功

Eighteen Techniques of Training Gong (i.e., Gongfu). One of the well known martial Qigong sets.

Ling 靈

Means supernatural spirit.

Liu He 六合

Means "six combinations" or "six unifications."

Liu He Ba Fa 六合八法

Literally: six combinations eight methods. A style of Chinese internal martial art reportedly created by Chen, Bo (陳博) during the Song Dynasty (960-1280 A.D.) (宋朝).

Liu Shu 六書

The six classifications of Chinese characters.

Min 敏

It can mean "smart," "alert," "fast action," "acute reaction," and "sensitive feeling."

Mu 木

Wood. One of the Five Phases.

Nan Yue 南岳

Also called "Heng Shan" (衡山)(Heng Mountain), one of the five great mountains in China. Heng San is located in Hunan Province (湖南省).

Ni Wan Gong 泥丸宮

Dust pill, or dust pill palace. Qigong terminology for the brain.

Pao Quan 炮拳

One of the Five Fists (Wu Quan, 五拳) in Xingyiquan.

Peng 鵬

A roc. A large legendary bird in China.

Pi Quan 劈拳

One of the Five Fists (Wu Quan, 五拳) in Xingyiquan.

Pu 撲

To leap. One of the strategic fighting actions in Xingyiquan.

Qi (Chi) 氣

The general definition of Qi is: universal energy, including heat, light, and electromagnetic energy. A narrower definition of Qi refers to the energy circulating in human or animal bodies.

Qi Xing 氣行

Means Qi transportation. The circulation of Qi.

Qi Xue 氣血

Literally: Qi-blood. Since blood cells are the carriers of Qi, Qi-blood are commonly used together in Chinese medicine.

Qian 乾

One of the Eight Trigrams which represents heaven.

Qigong (Chi Kung) 氣功

Gong (功) means Gongfu (功夫)(lit. energy-time). Therefore, Qigong means the study, research, and/or practices related to Qi.

Qihai (Co-6) 氣海

Means Qi ocean. An acupuncture cavities which is about one to two inches under the navel.

Qin Na (Chin Na) 擒拿

Literally, seize control. A type of Chinese Gongfu which emphasizes grabbing techniques to control the opponent's joints in conjunction with attacking certain acupuncture cavities. One of the main fighting categories in Chinese martial arts. These four categories are: kicking (Ti, 踢), striking (Da, 打), wrestling (Shuai, 摔), and controlling (Qin Na, 擒拿).

Qing Jing 清靜

Means cleanness and calmness. It implies the mind's peaceful and calm state.

Qingcheng Mountain 青城山

A mountain located in Sichuan Province (四川省).

Qu 曲

Means "to curve" or "to bend." One of the strategic fighting actions in Xingyiquan.

Quan 拳

Literally means "fist," but is also can mean "style" or "technique."

Ren 人

Man. One of the Three Powers (San Cai, 三才). Three Powers are: Heaven, Earth, and Man.

Ren Mai 任脈

Conception Vessel. One of the Eight Extraordinary Vessels in Chinese medicine and Qigong.

Renzhong (Gv-26) 人中

Means men's center. An acupuncture cavity which is located under the nose and above the upper lip.

Rou 肉

Meat and implies muscles and tendons in human body.

San Cai 三才

The "Three Powers: "Heaven (Tian, 天), Earth (Di, 地), and Man (Ren, 人).

San Guan 三關

Three Gates. Three obstacles in Small Circulation meditation practice. These three gates are: Weilu (尾閭)(i.e., tailbone), Jiaji (夾脊)(i.e., Squeeze Spine between shoulder blades), and Yuzhen (玉枕)(i.e., jade pillow).

San Ti Shi 三體式

Three Body Posture. The beginning posture of Xingyiquan.

Shanxi 陝西

A province in China.

Shang Dan Tian 上丹田

Upper Dan Tian (i.e., upper elixir field) which means "brain."

Shao 梢

The end of anything is called "Shao."

Shaolin 少林

A Buddhist temple in Henan Province (河南省), famous for its martial arts.

Shen Ning 神寧

Means the spirit is calm and peaceful.

Shi Er Jing 十二經

Twelve Primary Qi Channels in Chinese medicine.

Shi Er Xing 十二形

Twelve Shapes. Name of an advanced Xingyiquan sequence.

Shi Er Xing Gun 十二形棍

Twelve Shape Staff. Name of an advanced Xingyiquan sequence.

Shi Er Xing Qiang 十二形槍

Twelve Shape Spear. Name of an advanced Xingyiquan sequence.

Shi Ji 史記

The Historical Record by Si, Ma-Qian (司馬遷), one of the Dynastic Historical Books of China.

Shu 束

Means to bind or to seal. One of strategic fighting actions in Xingyiquan.

Shuai Jiao 摔跤

Chinese wrestling.

Shui 水

Water. One of the Five Phases.

Shun 順

Smoothness. One of the training requirements in Xingyiquan practice.

Si Shao 四梢

The four extremities which include tongue, teeth, nails, and hair.

Si Xiang 四象

Four Phases.

Sun Zi Bing Fa 孫子兵法

Sun's Book of Tactics, by Sun, Wu (c. 557 B.C.)(孫武)

Ta Qi Xing 踏七星

Means "stepping seven stars." A strategic stepping in Xingyiquan.

Taiji 太極

Means "grand ultimate." According to Chinese philosophy, Taiji is an invisible force which is able to make Wuji (無極)(i.e., no extremity) derived into Yin and Yang two poles and also vise versa.

Taiji Qigong 太極氣功

A Qigong practice based on Taiji theory.

Taijiquan 太極拳

Great ultimate fist. An internal style of Chinese martial art which is created based on the theory of Taiji.

Tang Lang 螳螂

Praying Mantis. An external style of Chinese martial art.

Teng 藤

Rattan.

Teng Pai Jun 藤牌軍

The Rattan Shield Army. A special military unit which was created by Marshal Yue, Fei (岳飛) to against Guai Zi Ma (拐子馬) during Chinese Southern Song Dynasty (1127-1280 A.D.).

Ti 提

Means to hold up.

Tian 天

Heaven. One of the Three Powers (San Cai, 三才).

Tian Yan 天眼

Literally: the heaven eye. It is equivalent to the third eye or Yintang (M-NH-3)(印堂) cavity in acupuncture.

Tianting 天庭

Literally: the heaven yard which is the Daoist name for the forehead.

Tiao Ling 挑領

Means to pluck and lead. One of the strategic fighting action in Xingyiquan.

Ting 挺

Means to stand up right, rigid, firm and strong, straightened, or thrust out.

Tou Quan 頭拳

Means the head punch (i.e., hand strikes). It is called this because the hand is the "head" of the punch.

Tu 土

Earth. One of the Five Phases.

Tui 退

Means to retreat or to get out of a disadvantageous position.

Tui Na 推拿

Literally: push and grab. Name of Chinese healing massage.

Wai Dan 外丹

External elixir. External Qigong exercises in which Qi is built up in the limbs and then led to the body.

Wei 渭

A river in Shanxi Province (陝西省).

Weilu 尾閭

Tailbone and is called Changqiang (Co-1, 長強) in Chinese acupuncture.

Wu Dao 五道

Five paths. Since the five paths are considered as the five gates which the opponent is able to enter, they may be the face, chest, abdomen, groin, and shin, which are the five common zones for an attack. However, it may imply the five directions which the enemy may enter, the front, rear, left, right, and center.

Wu Qi Chao Yuan 五氣朝元

Five Qi's toward origins. A goal of Qigong wherein the Qi of the five Yin organs (Heart, Lungs, Liver, Kidneys, and Spleen) is kept at the right (original) level. This will keep the organs from being either too Yang or too Yin, and will slow the degeneration process.

Wu Quan 五拳

"Five Fists." Also called "Wu Xing" (Five Phases), the five basic techniques of Xingyiquan.

Wu Wu 無物

Means "nothingness."

Wu Xing 五行

Five Phases which includes: Metal (Jin, 金), Wood (Mu, 木), Water (Shui, 水), Fire (Huo, 火), and Earth (Tu, 土).

Wu Xing Dao 五形刀

Five Shape Saber. One of the advanced Xingyiquan training sequences.

Wu Xing Jian 五形劍

Five Shape Sword. One of the advanced Xingyiquan training sequences.

Wu Xing Lian Huan Quan 五行連環拳

Five Phases Linking Sequence. A barehand training sequence for Xingyiquan beginners. This sequence is constructed by Five Fist (Wu Quan, 五拳).

Wu Xing Pao 五行炮

Five Phases Strike. One of the advanced Xingyiquan training sequences.

Wudang Mountain 武當山

Located in Fubei Province (湖北省) in China.

Wuji 無極

Means "no poles," and refers to the state where nothing is distinguished from anything else.

Wushu 武術

Literally: martial techniques. A common name for the Chinese martial arts. Many other terms are used, including: Wuyi (武藝)(martial arts), Wugong (武功)(martial Gongfu), Guoshu (國術)(national techniques), and Gongfu (功夫)(energy-time). Because Wushu has been modified in mainland China over the past forty years into gymnastic martial performance, many traditional Chinese martial artist have given up this name in order to avoid confusing modern Wushu with traditional Wushu. Recently, mainland China has attempted to bring modern Wushu back toward its traditional training and practice.

Xi Hu 西湖

West Lake in Hangzhou (杭州) of Zhejiang Province (浙江省).

Xi Sui Jing 洗髓經

Washing Marrow/Brain Classic, usually translated *Marrow/Brain Washing Classic.* Qigong training specializing in leading Qi to the marrow to cleanse it.

Xian Tian 先天

Pre-Heaven. It means before the birth.

Xiao Jiu Tian 小九天

Small Nine Heaven. A Qigong style created in the sixth century.

Xin 心

Literally: Heart. Refers to the emotional mind.

Xin An 心安

Means the emotional mind is peaceful.

Xin Ding 心定

Means the emotional mind is stabilized and calm.

Xin Wo 心窩

Means solar plexus area.

Xin Yi Quan 心意拳

Xingyiquan is also called Xin Yi Quan (i.e., the fist of Xin and Yi) because the heart (emotional mind) and Yi play an important role in the style.

Xing 形

Shape. The external appearance.

Xingyi 形意

Literally: Shape Mind. An aberration of Xingyiquan.

Xingyiquan (Xingyi) 形意拳

Literally: Shape-mind Fist. An internal style of Gongfu in which the mind or thinking determines the shape or movement of the body. Creation of the style attributed to Marshal Yue, Fei (岳飛).

Yan Shen 眼神

Eye spirit.

Yang 養

Means to nourish, to increase, to raise, and to cultivate.

Yang 陽

In Chinese philosophy, the active, positive, masculine polarity. In Chinese medicine, Yang means excessive, overactive, overheated.

Yang Qi 養氣

To refine, nurse, and nourish the Qi.

Yi 意

Mind. (Pronounced "ee") Specifically, the mind which is generated by clear thinking and judgement, and which is able to make you calm, peaceful, and wise.

Yi Gong Wei Shou 以攻為守

One of the Chinese martial arts strategies which uses attack as the defense.

Yi Jin Jing 易筋經

Literally: *Changing Muscle/Tendon Classic*, usually called *The Muscle/Tendon Changing Classic*. Credited to Da Mo around 550 A.D., this work discusses Wai Dan Qigong (外丹氣功) training for strengthening the physical body.

Yi Jing 易經

Book of Changes. An ancient book written about four thousand years ago.

Yin 陰

In Chinese philosophy, the passive, negative, feminine polarity. In Chinese medicine, Yin means deficient. The Yin (internal) organs are the Heart, Lungs, Liver, Kidneys, Spleen, and Pericardium.

Ying Zhuo 鷹捉

Literally: eagle's seizing.

Yintang (M-NH-3) 印堂

An acupuncture cavity which is the third eye area.

Yongquan (K-1) 湧泉

An acupuncture cavity which is located at the bottom of feet.

Yuan 圓

Round.

Yuan Jing 元精

Original Essence. The fundamental, original substance inherited from your parents, it is converted into Original Qi (元氣).

Yuan Qi 元氣

Original Qi. Created from the Original Essence inherited from your parents.

Yuan Shen 元神

Original Spirit. The spirit you already had when you were born.

Yue Jia Jun 岳家軍

Yue Family Troop. The troop led by Marshal Yue, Fei (岳飛).

Yue Jia Ying Zhua 岳家鷹爪

Yue Family's Eagle Claw. A martial style which was created by Marshal Yue, Fei.

Yue Wu Mu 岳武穆

"Yue, the righteous and respectable warrior." A title given to Marshal Yue, Fei by Emperor Xiao Zong (孝宗) in 1166 A.D.

Yue, Fei 岳飛

A famous Chinese hero during the Southern Song Dynasty (南宋)(1127-1280 A.D.).

Yuzhen 玉枕

Jade pillow. One of the three gates of Small Circulation training.

Zhan Shou 沾手

Sticky hands. The skills commonly used in short range fighting especially in internal styles.

Zhang, San-Feng 張三豐

A Daoist credited with creating Taijiquan during the Song Dynasty (960-1280 A.D.)(宋朝).

Zhang, Xiang-San 張祥三

A well-known Chinese martial artist in Taiwan during 1960's.

Zhong Men 中門

Literally: center door, which is right in front of the opponent's chest.

Zhongtang 中堂

Means the center of the face.

Zhongwan (Co-12) 中脘

An acupuncture cavity around stomach area.

Zuan 鑽

Means to drill. One of the strategic fighting skills in Xingyiquan.

Zuan Bu 躦步

Drill stepping. One of the strategic stepping in Xingyiquan.

Zuan Quan 劈拳

One of the Five Fist (Wu Quan, 五拳).

Index

101 REFLECTIONS ON TAI CHI CHUAN
108 INSIGHTS INTO TAI CHI CHUAN
A WOMAN'S QIGONG GUIDE
ADVANCING IN TAE KWON DO
ANALYSIS OF GENUINE KARATE
ANALYSIS OF GENUINE KARATE 2
ANALYSIS OF SHAOLIN CHIN NA 2ND ED
ANCIENT CHINESE WEAPONS
ART AND SCIENCE OF STAFF FIGHTING
THE ART AND SCIENCE OF SELF-DEFENSE
ART AND SCIENCE OF STICK FIGHTING
ART OF HOJO UNDO
ARTHRITIS RELIEF
BACK PAIN RELIEF
BAGUAZHANG
BRAIN FITNESS
CHIN NA IN GROUND FIGHTING
CHINESE FAST WRESTLING
CHINESE FITNESS
CHINESE TUI NA MASSAGE
COMPLETE MARTIAL ARTIST
COMPREHENSIVE APPLICATIONS OF SHAOLIN CHIN NA
CONFLICT COMMUNICATION
DAO DE JING: A QIGONG INTERPRETATION
DAO IN ACTION
DEFENSIVE TACTICS
DIRTY GROUND
DR. WU'S HEAD MASSAGE
ESSENCE OF SHAOLIN WHITE CRANE
EXPLORING TAI CHI
FACING VIOLENCE
FIGHT LIKE A PHYSICIST
THE FIGHTER'S BODY
FIGHTER'S FACT BOOK 1&2
FIGHTING THE PAIN RESISTANT ATTACKER
FIRST DEFENSE
FORCE DECISIONS: A CITIZENS GUIDE
INSIDE TAI CHI
JUDO ADVANTAGE
JUJI GATAME ENCYCLOPEDIA
KARATE SCIENCE
KEPPAN
KRAV MAGA COMBATIVES
KRAV MAGA FUNDAMENTAL STRATEGIES
KRAV MAGA PROFESSIONAL TACTICS
KRAV MAGA WEAPON DEFENSES
LITTLE BLACK BOOK OF VIOLENCE
LIUHEBAFA FIVE CHARACTER SECRETS
MARTIAL ARTS OF VIETNAM
MARTIAL ARTS INSTRUCTION
MARTIAL WAY AND ITS VIRTUES
MEDITATIONS ON VIOLENCE
MERIDIAN QIGONG EXERCISES
MINDFUL EXERCISE
MIND INSIDE TAI CHI
MIND INSIDE YANG STYLE TAI CHI CHUAN
NORTHERN SHAOLIN SWORD
OKINAWA'S COMPLETE KARATE SYSTEM: ISSHIN RYU
PRINCIPLES OF TRADITIONAL CHINESE MEDICINE
PROTECTOR ETHIC
QIGONG FOR HEALTH & MARTIAL ARTS
QIGONG FOR TREATING COMMON AILMENTS

QIGONG MASSAGE
QIGONG MEDITATION: EMBRYONIC BREATHING
QIGONG GRAND CIRCULATION
QIGONG MEDITATION: SMALL CIRCULATION
QIGONG, THE SECRET OF YOUTH: DA MO'S CLASSICS
ROOT OF CHINESE QIGONG
SAMBO ENCYCLOPEDIA
SCALING FORCE
SELF-DEFENSE FOR WOMEN
SHIN GI TAI: KARATE TRAINING
SIMPLE CHINESE MEDICINE
SIMPLE QIGONG EXERCISES FOR HEALTH, 3RD ED.
SIMPLIFIED TAI CHI CHUAN, 2ND ED.
SOLO TRAINING 1&2
SPOTTING DANGER BEFORE IT SPOTS YOU
SPOTTING DANGER BEFORE IT SPOTS YOUR KIDS
SPOTTING DANGER BEFORE IT SPOTS YOUR TEENS
SPOTTING DANGER FOR TRAVELERS
SUMO FOR MIXED MARTIAL ARTS
SUNRISE TAI CHI
SURVIVING ARMED ASSAULTS
TAE KWON DO: THE KOREAN MARTIAL ART
TAEKWONDO BLACK BELT POOMSAE
TAEKWONDO: A PATH TO EXCELLENCE
TAEKWONDO: ANCIENT WISDOM
TAEKWONDO: DEFENSE AGAINST WEAPONS
TAEKWONDO: SPIRIT AND PRACTICE
TAI CHI BALL QIGONG: FOR HEALTH AND MARTIAL ARTS
TAI CHI BALL QIGONG
THE TAI CHI BOOK
TAI CHI CHIN NA
TAI CHI CHUAN CLASSICAL YANG STYLE
TAI CHI CHUAN MARTIAL APPLICATIONS
TAI CHI CHUAN MARTIAL POWER
TAI CHI CONCEPTS AND EXPERIMENTS
TAI CHI DYNAMICS
TAI CHI FOR DEPRESSION
TAI CHI IN 10 WEEKS
TAI CHI PUSH HANDS
TAI CHI QIGONG
TAI CHI SECRETS OF THE ANCIENT MASTERS
TAI CHI SECRETS OF THE WU & LI STYLES
TAI CHI SECRETS OF THE WU STYLE
TAI CHI SECRETS OF THE YANG STYLE
TAI CHI SWORD: CLASSICAL YANG STYLE
TAI CHI SWORD FOR BEGINNERS
TAI CHI WALKING
TAI CHI CHUAN THEORY OF DR. YANG, JWING-MING
FIGHTING ARTS
TRADITIONAL CHINESE HEALTH SECRETS
TRADITIONAL TAEKWONDO
TRAINING FOR SUDDEN VIOLENCE
TRIANGLE HOLD ENCYCLOPEDIA
TRUE WELLNESS SERIES (MIND, HEART, GUT)
WARRIOR'S MANIFESTO
WAY OF KATA
WAY OF SANCHIN KATA
WAY TO BLACK BELT
WESTERN HERBS FOR MARTIAL ARTISTS
WILD GOOSE QIGONG
WING CHUN IN-DEPTH
WINNING FIGHTS
XINGYIQUAN

AND MANY MORE . . .

VIDEOS FROM YMAA

ANALYSIS OF SHAOLIN CHIN NA
ART AND SCIENCE OF SELF DEFENSE
ART AND SCIENCE OF STAFF FIGHTING
ART AND SCIENCE STICK FIGHTING
BAGUA FOR BEGINNERS 1 & 2
BAGUAZHANG: EMEI BAGUAZHANG
BEGINNER QIGONG FOR WOMEN 1 & 2
BEGINNER TAI CHI FOR HEALTH
BREATH MEDICINE
BIOENERGY TRAINING 1&2
CHEN TAI CHI CANNON FIST
CHEN TAI CHI FIRST FORM
CHEN TAI CHI FOR BEGINNERS
CHIN NA IN-DEPTH SERIES
FACING VIOLENCE: 7 THINGS A MARTIAL ARTIST MUST KNOW
FIVE ANIMAL SPORTS
FIVE ELEMENTS ENERGY BALANCE
HEALER WITHIN: MEDICAL QIGONG
INFIGHTING
INTRODUCTION TO QI GONG FOR BEGINNERS
JOINT LOCKS
KNIFE DEFENSE
KUNG FU BODY CONDITIONING 1 & 2
KUNG FU FOR KIDS AND TEENS SERIES
MERIDIAN QIGONG
NEIGONG FOR MARTIAL ARTS
NORTHERN SHAOLIN SWORD
QI GONG 30-DAY CHALLENGE
QI GONG FOR ANXIETY
QI GONG FOR ARMS, WRISTS, AND HANDS
QIGONG FOR BEGINNERS: FRAGRANCE
QI GONG FOR BETTER BALANCE
QI GONG FOR BETTER BREATHING
QI GONG FOR CANCER
QI GONG FOR DEPRESSION
QI GONG FOR ENERGY AND VITALITY
QI GONG FOR HEADACHES
QIGONG FOR HEALTH: HEALING QIGONG
QIGONG FOR HEALTH: IMMUNE SYSTEM
QI GONG FOR THE HEALTHY HEART
QI GONG FOR HEALTHY JOINTS
QI GONG FOR HIGH BLOOD PRESSURE
QIGONG FOR LONGEVITY
QI GONG FOR STRONG BONES
QI GONG FOR THE UPPER BACK AND NECK
QIGONG FOR WOMEN WITH DAISY LEE
QIGONG FLOW FOR STRESS & ANXIETY RELIEF
QIGONG GRAND CIRCULATION
QIGONG MASSAGE
QIGONG MINDFULNESS IN MOTION
QI GONG—THE SEATED WORKOUT
QIGONG: 15 MINUTES TO HEALTH
SABER FUNDAMENTAL TRAINING
SAI TRAINING AND SEQUENCES
SANCHIN KATA: TRADITIONAL TRAINING FOR KARATE POWER
SCALING FORCE
SEARCHING FOR SUPERHUMANS
SHAOLIN KUNG FU FUNDAMENTAL TRAINING: COURSES 1 & 2
SHAOLIN LONG FIST KUNG FU BEGINNER—INTERMEDIATE—
    ADVANCED SERIES
SHAOLIN SABER: BASIC SEQUENCES
SHAOLIN STAFF: BASIC SEQUENCES
SHAOLIN WHITE CRANE GONG FU BASIC TRAINING SERIES

SHUAI JIAO: KUNG FU WRESTLING
SIMPLE QIGONG EXERCISES FOR HEALTH
SIMPLE QIGONG EXERCISES FOR ARTHRITIS RELIEF
SIMPLE QIGONG EXERCISES FOR BACK PAIN RELIEF
SIMPLIFIED TAI CHI CHUAN: 24 & 48 POSTURES
SIMPLIFIED TAI CHI FOR BEGINNERS 48
SPOTTING DANGER BEFORE IT SPOTS YOU
SPOTTING DANGER FOR KIDS
SPOTTING DANGER FOR TEENS
SUN TAI CHI
SWORD: FUNDAMENTAL TRAINING
TAEKWONDO KORYO POOMSAE
TAI CHI BALL QIGONG SERIES
TAI CHI BALL WORKOUT FOR BEGINNERS
TAI CHI CHUAN CLASSICAL YANG STYLE
TAI CHI FIGHTING SET
TAI CHI FIT: 24 FORM
TAI CHI FIT: ALZHEIMER'S PREVENTION
TAI CHI FIT: CANCER PREVENTION
TAI CHI FIT FOR VETERANS
TAI CHI FIT: FOR WOMEN
TAI CHI FIT: FLOW
TAI CHI FIT: FUSION BAMBOO
TAI CHI FIT: FUSION FIRE
TAI CHI FIT: FUSION IRON
TAI CHI FIT: HEALTHY BACK SEATED WORKOUT
TAI CHI FIT: HEALTHY HEART WORKOUT
TAI CHI FIT IN PARADISE
TAI CHI FIT: OVER 50
TAI CHI FIT OVER 50: BALANCE EXERCISES
TAI CHI FIT OVER 50: SEATED WORKOUT
TAI CHI FIT OVER 60: GENTLE EXERCISES
TAI CHI FIT OVER 60: HEALTHY JOINTS
TAI CHI FIT OVER 60: LIVE LONGER
TAI CHI FIT: STRENGTH
TAI CHI FIT: TO GO
TAI CHI FOR WOMEN
TAI CHI FUSION: FIRE
TAI CHI QIGONG
TAI CHI PRINCIPLES FOR HEALTHY AGING
TAI CHI PUSHING HANDS SERIES
TAI CHI SWORD: CLASSICAL YANG STYLE
TAI CHI SWORD FOR BEGINNERS
TAI CHI SYMBOL: YIN YANG STICKING HANDS
TAIJI & SHAOLIN STAFF: FUNDAMENTAL TRAINING
TAIJI CHIN NA IN-DEPTH
TAIJI 37 POSTURES MARTIAL APPLICATIONS
TAIJI SABER CLASSICAL YANG STYLE
TAIJI WRESTLING
TRAINING FOR SUDDEN VIOLENCE
UNDERSTANDING QIGONG SERIES
WATER STYLE FOR BEGINNERS
WHITE CRANE HARD & SOFT QIGONG
YANG TAI CHI FOR BEGINNERS
YOQI: MICROCOSMIC ORBIT QIGONG
YOQI QIGONG FOR A HAPPY HEART
YOQI:QIGONG FLOW FOR HAPPY MIND
YOQI:QIGONG FLOW FOR INTERNAL ALCHEMY
YOQI QIGONG FOR HAPPY SPLEEN & STOMACH
YOQI QIGONG FOR HAPPY KIDNEYS
YOQI QIGONG FLOW FOR HAPPY LUNGS
YOQI QIGONG FLOW FOR STRESS RELIEF
YOQI: QIGONG FLOW TO BOOST IMMUNE SYSTEM

more products available from . . .
YMAA Publication Center, Inc. 楊氏東方文化出版中心
1-800-669-8892 • info@ymaa.com • www.ymaa.com

YMAA
PUBLICATION CENTER

www.ingramcontent.com/pod-product-compliance
Lightning Source LLC
Chambersburg PA
CBHW080756300326
41914CB00055B/912